EYE AND VISION RESEARCH DEVELOPMENTS

# MACULAR EDEMA

# RISK FACTORS, TREATMENT OPTIONS AND LONG-TERM OUTCOMES

# EYE AND VISION RESEARCH DEVELOPMENTS

Additional books in this series can be found on Nova's website under the Series tab.

Additional e-books in this series can be found on Nova's website under the e-book tab.

EYE AND VISION RESEARCH DEVELOPMENTS

# MACULAR EDEMA

## RISK FACTORS, TREATMENT OPTIONS AND LONG-TERM OUTCOMES

EARL DAVISON

EDITOR

nova publishers

*New York*

For permission to use material from this book please contact us:
Telephone 631-231-7269; Fax 631-231-8175
Web Site: http://www.novapublishers.com



**Library of Congress Cataloging-in-Publication Data**

ISBN: 978-1-63321-584-9
Library of Congress Control Number: 2014945324

*Published by Nova Science Publishers, Inc. † New York*

# CONTENTS

# PREFACE

Macular edema is a serious eye disorder that can be seen in many conditions. Central retinal vein occlusion (CRVO) and branch retinal vein occlusion (BRVO) are frequent causes of decreased central visual acuity (VA) related to the appearance of macular edema (ME) and ischemia. This book discusses the risk factors, treatment options and long-term outcomes of macular edema. Some of the topics discussed include the management of diabetic macular edema; management of macular edema secondary to retinal vein occulsion by intravitreal bevacizumab; and macular edema in important tropical infections.

Chapter 1 – The definition, classification and management of diabetic macular edema (DME) have changed during the past two decades due to the advent of optical coherence tomography and the new intravitreal treatments. Intravitreal anti vascular endothelial growth factor (VEGF) therapies have become indispensable tools in the management of DME as monotherapy or combined with intravitreal steroids, laser photocoagulation and surgery. However, these treatments are also associated with potentially severe local and systemic side effects. Presently, four different intravitreal anti-VEGF drugs are available (one of them as an off-label treatment). Comparative clinical trials have been performed on the efficacy of these treatments and even though some of these drugs have proved to exert a similar effect in randomized clinical trials on age related macular degeneration, there seems to be more differences in DME. Presently there is an ongoing study to evaluate the comparative effectiveness of intravitreal aflibercept, bevacizumab, and ranibizumab for DME. In the present chapter the authors discuss the pros and cons of the different treatments as well as their respective indications, with a revision of the clinical evidence and trials as well as the authors' personal experience. Treatment algorithms are proposed.

Chapter 2 – Central retinal vein occlusion (CRVO) and branch retinal vein occlusion (BRVO) are frequent causes of decreased central visual acuity (VA) related to the appearance of macular edema (ME) and ischemia. Laser treatment does not seem to improve final VA in CRVO. High intravitreous levels of vascular endothelial growth factor (VEGF) have been reported and therefore, intravitreous anti VEGF drugs have been used in an attempt to improve visual and anatomic outcome. Recent clinical trials have revealed the efficacy of intravitreous therapy with ranibizumab and aflibercept to reduce ME improving VA, and these drugs have been approved for such indication. Several series have reported on the efficacy of off-label intravitreous bevacizumab (IVB) to manage ME. The visual and anatomical outcome and treatment regimes of IVB in the management of ME secondary to retinal vein occlusion are discussed and compared with those results previously reported in the literature as well as the results of the main clinical trials performed with other intravitreous anti VEGF drugs.

Chapter 3 – The risk of cataracts among diabetic patients is three to five-fold higher than that of healthy population and uneventful phacoemulsification is sometimes associated with an increased risk of aggravation of diabetic retinopathy and macular edema. These increased risks have been related to an over-expression of inflammatory mediators, especially of vascular endothelial growth factor (VEGF). Postoperative macular edema may resolve spontaneously, but most frequently it will reduce the expected visual acuity improvement. Among the most usual strategies for the prevention of postoperative macular edema in diabetic patients, preoperative laser photocoagulation and intra operative intravitreal steroids and anti-VEGF drugs have been advocated. Similarly, it has been suggested that topical anti-inflammatory drops may improve visual outcome after surgery. Nd-YAG laser treatment of postoperative posterior capsular opacification can also be linked to an increased risk of macular edema. Spectral Domain Optical Coherence Tomography is a very sensitive tool for the identification of macular changes associated with surgery. In this chapter the authors revise the most usual strategies for the prophylaxis and management of postoperative macular edema in diabetic patients as well as their experience and the results of the most recent clinical trials.

Chapter 4 – Diabetic macular edema (DME) is the main cause of visual impairment in patients with diabetes mellitus (DM). For many years macular laser photocoagulation has been the golf standard therapy for preventing severe visual loss in patients with DME. However, intravitreal pharmacological therapies have changed how DME is managed, improving visual function with a well-documented tolerable safety profile, and providing patients with significant visual acuity gains that are sustainable with repeat injections. Thus, it has been proposed the use of anti-VEGF or corticosteroids agents as the first line of treatment instead of laser therapy in patients with center-involving DME with moderate visual impairment. Patients who do not yet meet the treatment threshold should be managed with laser therapy according to ETDRS guidelines. On the other hand, although further researches are necessary to establish the best way to care DME patients, and given its multifactorial nature, combination therapy of anti-VEGF drugs with corticosteroids is an evolving field in an effort to alleviate the treatment burden of monthly dosing and to assess the efficacy in those individuals with persistent DME despite repeated anti-VEGF injections.

Chapter 5 – Diabetic macular oedema (DMO) is a leading cause of visual impairment in people with diabetes mellitus. Defined as retinal thickening involving or approaching the center of the macula, if left untreated more than half of patients lose more than two lines of visual acuity within 2 years. DMO results in a significant socioeconomic burden, particularly affecting the working-age population. This burden will increase in parallel with the inexorable rise in the prevalence of diabetes globally. A thorough understanding of the pathogenesis of chronic DMO is required to delineate the functional and clinical characteristics of the disease. Furthermore, for effective management of the condition, a multidisciplinary approach is necessary with intervention at both systemic and local levels. Treatment for DMO is continuously evolving with the advent of novel pharmacologic therapies. Despite this, focal laser photocoagulation remains the mainstay of treatment. Data from the most recent clinical trials of therapies for this complex condition have confirmed the benefit of intravitreal antivascular endothelial growth factor (anti-VEGF) medications and corticosteroids. The aim of this review is to provide an overview of current treatment perspectives by discussing the various treatment options for chronic DMO.

Chapter 6 – There are many problematic tropical infections at present. The good examples include dengue, malaria, etc. Those infections can have the ophthalmological presentations. The ophthalmological presentations might be difficult to diagnose and easily forgotten. This might bring several unwanted outcome. The macular edema is a serious eye disorder that can be seen in many conditions including to the tropical infections. In this specific short article, the authors summarize on important tropical infections and the relating problems of macular edema. The discussion will cover the risk, treatment, complication and outcome of those macular edema disorders in present clinical practice.

Chapter 7 – This article is concerned with the problem of treating cystoid macular edema. The various methods of treating macular edema are briefly described and then a case report on a patient, the author, is presented. The author developed cystoid macular edema following an operation to cure a macular hole by vitrectomy. Four treatments were applied. All were successful to some degree but none abolished the edema. Details of two treatments, anti-inflammatory eye-drops and acetazolamide (a carbonic anhydrase inhibitor), will not be presented. The other two treatments, hyperbaric oxygen and estrogen, are described in moderate detail and the reason why macular edema is so difficult to treat is discussed in some detail. Suggestions are made as to how the research should proceed.

In: Macular Edema
Editor: Earl Davison

ISBN: 978-1-63321-584-9


*Chapter 1*

# MANAGEMENT OF DIABETIC MACULAR EDEMA BY INTRAVITREAL ANTIANGIOGENIC DRUGS

***Javier A. Montero-Moreno*[1,2], *Jose M. Ruiz-Moreno*[3,4], *Rosa M. Sanabria-Colmenares*[5] *and Marta Fernandez-Muñoz*[1]**

[1]Pio del Rio Hortega University Hospital, Valladolid, Spain
[2]Retina Unit, Oftalvist Moncloa, Madrid, Spain
[3]Department of Ophthalmology, Castilla La Mancha University, Albacete, Spain
[4]Baviera Clinic, European Opthalmic Institute, Alicante, Spain
[5]Palencia Hospital, Palencia, Spain

## ABSTRACT

The definition, classification and management of diabetic macular edema (DME) have changed during the past two decades due to the advent of optical coherence tomography and the new intravitreal treatments. Intravitreal anti vascular endothelial growth factor (VEGF) therapies have become indispensable tools in the management of DME as monotherapy or combined with intravitreal steroids, laser photocoagulation and surgery. However, these treatments are also associated with potentially severe local and systemic side effects.

Presently, four different intravitreal anti-VEGF drugs are available (one of them as an off-label treatment). Comparative clinical trials have been performed on the efficacy of these treatments and even though some of these drugs have proved to exert a similar effect in randomized clinical trials on age related macular degeneration, there seems to be more differences in DME. Presently there is an ongoing study to evaluate the comparative effectiveness of intravitreal aflibercept, bevacizumab, and ranibizumab for DME.

In the present chapter we discuss the pros and cons of the different treatments as well as their respective indications, with a revision of the clinical evidence and trials as well as our personal experience. Treatment algorithms are proposed.

## INTRODUCTION

Diabetic macular edema (DME) is a frequent ocular complication of diabetes mellitus (DM) and the leading cause of central vision and visual acuity (VA) loss among diabetic patients. DME results from microvascular changes occurring in the retina in DM type 1 and 2. Legal blindness in DM type 2 patients is most frequently caused by DME, and its prevalence is directly correlated to the duration of DM.

DME is defined by retinal thickening of an area comprised within 1 disk diameter from the fovea; DME located within or close to the central macula is termed clinically significant macular edema (CSME). DME can be classified in terms of its pathogenic mechanism as focal DME (caused by fluid leakage from individual micro aneurysms) (Figure 1) and diffuse DME (secondary to extensive or generalized leakage from the posterior capillary bed and breakdown of the inner blood-retinal bed) (Figures 2, 3), and is frequently caused by a combination of both mechanisms.

DR affects between 25% and 44% of diabetic patients. Eight well-conducted population-based studies showed an overall prevalence of DR of 40% with a prevalence of sight-threatening retinopathy (CSME and proliferative diabetic retinopathy, PDR) of 8.2% [1].

The most frequent first presentation of DME is blurred vision and distortion of central vision (metamorphopsia), combined with decreased contrast sensitivity, photophobia, changes in color vision and scotoma.

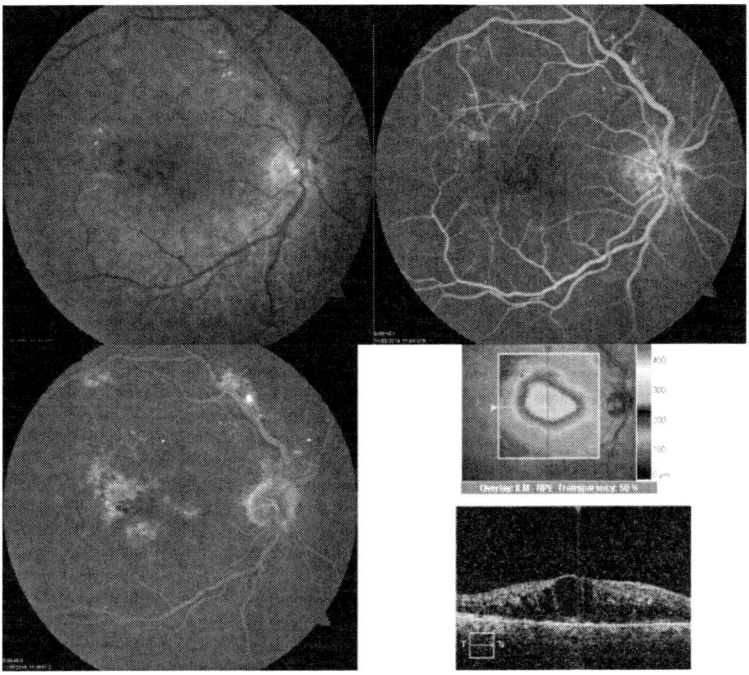

Figure 1. Fundus photograph and fluorescein angiography of an eye with focal diabetic macular edema.

DME and CSME can be evaluated by slit lamp biomicroscopy, or by grading stereo photographs of the posterior segment. Fluorescein angiography (FA) permits a proper assessment of the leaking points and optical coherence tomography (OCT) provides a useful confirmation and quantification of retinal thickening, facilitating an objective monitoring of the clinical response to treatment.

The pathogenesis of diabetic retinopathy (DR) is mediated by an inflammatory process in which leukocyte adhesion, cytokine cascades and varied growth factors such as the vascular endothelial growth factor (VEGF) play a key role. The intercellular endothelial-endothelial unions in the capillary bed are disorganized, leading to a breakdown of the blood-retinal barrier and the subsequent increased vascular permeability and appearance of pathologic retinal vascularization. Varied factors are involved in the pathogenesis of DME. DME is caused by a generalized breakdown of the inner blood-retinal barrier, leading to accumulation of fluid and plasma constituents, such as lipoproteins, within the intraretinal layers of the macula.

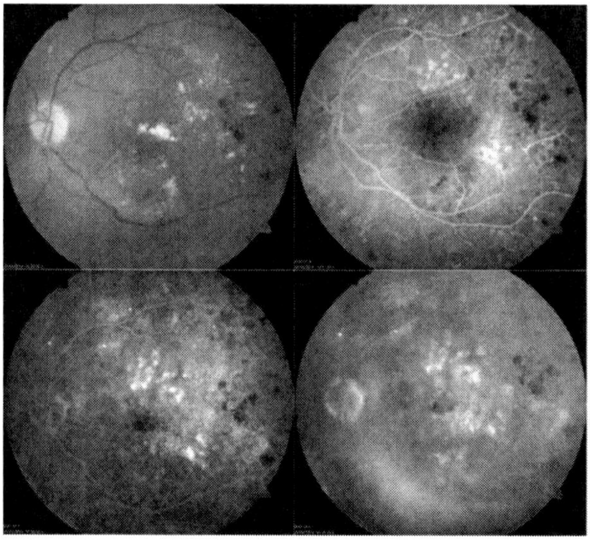

Figure 2. Fundus photograph and fluorescein angiography of an eye with diffuse diabetic macular edema, with multiple hard exudates and hemorrhages as well as non-perfused areas.

Retinal vascular leakage and ischemia are involved in a great part of the retinal damage. The most important part of prevention and management of this condition is a strict control of glycaemia, lypidemia and arterial pressure.

Presently, different therapeutic approaches have been proposed for the management of DME, even though none of them is completely satisfactory. Focal or grid laser photocoagulation have been used to destroy retinal tissue, and the Early Treatment Diabetic Retinopathy Study (ETDRS) proved its efficacy reducing the risk of moderate vision loss, becoming a standard treatment in clinical practice [2]. (Figure 4) Laser treatment is still a keystone of the management of DME, even though it may also cause visible scars that may expand causing decreased VA. Different macular laser treatment techniques have been proposed such as sub threshold micro pulse diode grid [3], temporal grid [4], minimal intensity diode laser photocoagulation [5], or subconjunctival triamcinolone acetonide (TA) assisted grid laser [6]. However, laser treatment is frequently unsuccessful especially in cases of chronic diffuse DME and implies creation of scotoma, what has led to an increased popularity of new surgical or medical therapies such as vitrectomy with removal of the posterior hyaloid or the inner limiting membrane, intravitreal steroids (TA, dexamethasone implants), anti angiogenic drugs or combined therapies.

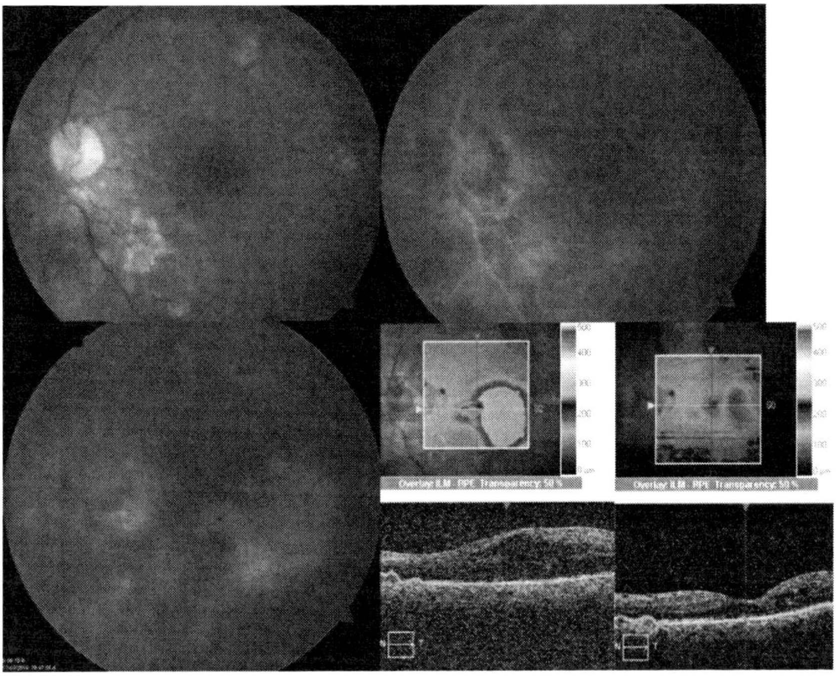

Figure 3. Fundus photograph and fluorescein angiography of an eye with diffuse diabetic macular edema.

Intravitreal TA causes a marked decrease of DME, and has been used at different concentrations [7-9]; however, its transient therapeutic effect combined with the frequent side effects (ocular hypertension and cataracts) have limited its use. Other steroids have been used with similar advantages and side effects [10]. VEGF up-regulation is associated in different ways with the pathogenesis of DME, so it seems reasonable to consider that VEGF inhibitors such as pegaptanib, ranibizumab, bevacizumab and aflibercept may be a promising strategy for the management of DME.

## Role of VEGF

The existence of a soluble angiogenesis factor causing ocular neovascularization was proposed by Michaelson [11]. Senger et al. described a molecule that altered the blood-brain and blood-retinal barriers [12], and called it vascular permeability factor; VEGF was discovered in 1989 [13, 14].

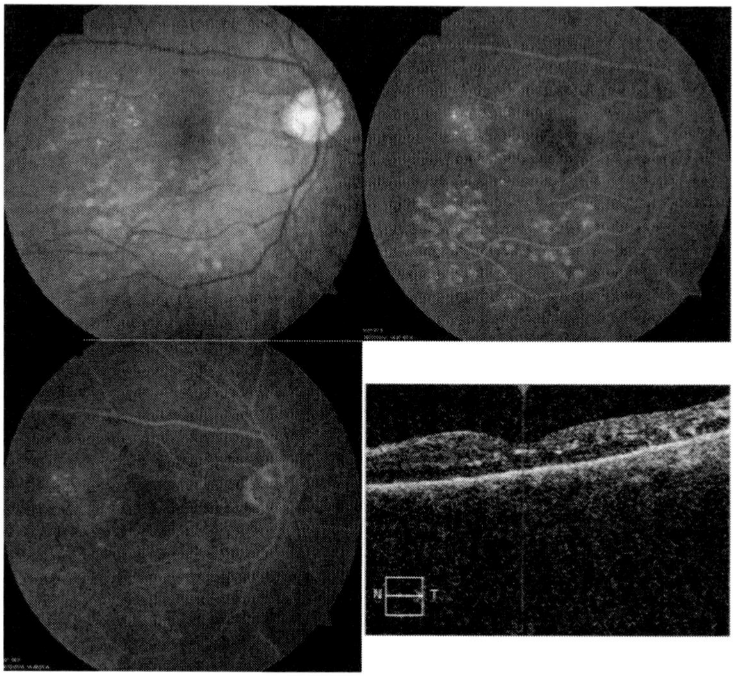


Figure 4. Fundus photograph and fluorescein angiography of an eye with focal diabetic macular edema that has been treated with grid photocoagulation.

Native VEGF (average molecular weight 35–45 kDa) is a mixture of several closely related homodimer glycoproteins that segregate into seven families: VEGFA, VEGFB, VEGFC, VEGFD, VEGFE, VEGFF, and placental growth factor (PlGF). Ocular neovascularization and increased vascular permeability occur when isoforms of VEGFA attach to the extracellular binding site of the transmembrane receptor, VEGFR2. Dimerization of the bound receptors induces conformational changes that activate the intracellular tyrosine kinase moieties on the receptors. Subsequent phosphorylation of target proteins up-regulate several downstream pathways, resulting in vascular endothelial cell proliferation and migration, activation of matrix metalloproteinases, breakdown of the blood-retinal barrier, vascular dilation, endothelial cell swelling, attraction of monocytes and macrophages, and attraction of endothelial cell precursors. VEGF has an important effect on the migration and mitosis of endothelial cells, up-regulating methane mono oxigenase and the creation of blood vessel lumen and fenestrations. VEFG plays a key role in the correct vascularization of the embryo or choroidal neovascularization, retinopathy of prematurity and tumor vascularization [15], and facilitates survival of existing vessels contributing to vascular abnormalities such as tortuousness and stimulates new vessel growth [16].

VEGF shows a pro-inflammatory effect and may intervene in the increased leukocyte adhesion to the new vessels. The intercellular adhesion molecule-1 (ICAM-1) and the vascular cell adhesion molecule-1 (VCAM-1) are regulated by VEGF among other molecules, and their over-expression causes increased leukocyte adhesion or leukostasis. Leukocyte adhesion causes an obstruction of retinal capillary vessels and a very slow leukocyte circulation, permitting an interaction between the endothelial cells and the leukocytes inducing endothelial damage, increased retinal vascular permeability, retinal edema and decreased VA. The obstruction of retinal capillaries increases retinal hypoxia and causes an over-expression of pro-angiogenic factors that will further aggravate the process.

Hypoxia-mediated VEGF release seems to intervene in the normal development of the retina. Expression of VEGF messenger ribonucleic acid shows a good spatial and temporal correlation with neovascularization in animal models of retinal ischemia [15], and high concentrations of VEGF have been reported in the aqueous and vitreous of human patients with ischemic and vasoproliferative conditions [17].

VEGF is involved in the breakdown of the blood-retinal barrier by phosphorylation of endothelial tight junction proteins, thus increasing vascular permeability. Vascular leakage from hypoxic retina is associated with intracellular edema of astrocytes and Müller's cells, breaking the unions of endothelial cells and the basal membrane of the internal blood-retinal barrier. Damage to the ionic homeostasis and production of free radicals during hypoxia-ischemia are responsible for intracellular edema. On the other hand, VEGF promotes the survival of vascular endothelial cells and neuroglia.

Anti-VEGF drugs seem to restore the integrity of the blood-retinal barrier, reducing retinal edema. Wang et al. reported on the down-regulation of VEGF and ICAM-1 expression in diabetic rats after intravitreal injection of dexamethasone, reducing leukocyte accumulation and retinal vascular permeability [18].

VEGF is over-expressed in the external segment of the photoreceptors, astrocytes and Müller's cells in the hypoxic retina. In the diabetic eye VEGF is secreted by the cells of the retinal pigment epithelium (RPE), pericytes and retinal endothelial cells in response to hypoxia [17]. The intravitreal concentration of VEGF is higher among diabetic patients than among non-diabetic patients, and is correlated to the hyper fluorescence level (in patients with non-proliferative DR and DME) [19]. Even after vitrectomy, eyes with

PDR show high intravitreal concentrations of VEGF, and these levels are higher than those found in peripheral blood, suggesting a local maintained production of VEGF [20]. These findings suggest that VEGF inhibition can play a significant role in the prophylaxis and management of diabetic ocular complications related to the appearance of microvascular damage.

The therapeutic effect of anti-VEGF drugs in the reduction of macular edema secondary to retinal vein occlusion and diabetic retinopathy, as well as its antiangiogenic effect in choroidal neovascularization secondary to age related macular degeneration and high myopia has been recently reported.

## PEGAPTANIB (MACUGEN®, PFIZER OPHTHALMICS)

Pegaptanib sodium (Macugen®, Eyetech Pharmaceuticals, Inc. and Pfizer Inc, New York) is a ribonucleic acid aptamer that targets the $VEGF_{165}$ isoform. Pegaptanib has a double mechanism as an antiangiogenic drug and preserving the blood-retinal barrier. It is highly specific for the $VEGF_{165}$ isoform, neutralizes the $VEGF_{164}$ isoform and does not induce an immune response. Intravitreal injection of pegaptanib does not influence plasma levels of VEGF [21]. It is intravitreally injected every 6 weeks and had a good safety profile in the clinical trials performed for exudative age related macular degeneration (AMD) and DME. Pegaptanib is currently approved in a number of countries worldwide for the treatment of exudative AMD [22].

However, despite the initial enthusiasm on the safety and results of this drug, its use in this indication was markedly reduced by the greater efficacy of other anti-VEGF drugs [23]. To date, eight clinical trials have been registered in the www.clinicaltrials.gov under the key words *DME* and *pegaptanib*, three of them with results. A phase II randomized, double-masked, multicenter, dose-ranging, controlled trial was performed in order to evaluate the safety and efficacy of pegaptanib in the treatment of DME [24]. One hundred seventy-two patients with VA between 65 and 25 letters and DME involving the center of the macula were included and randomized to be treated by intravitreous pegaptanib (0.3mg, 1mg, 3mg) or sham injections at week 0, week 6, and week 12 with additional injections and/or focal photocoagulation as needed for another 18 weeks.

At week 36 patients were evaluated for VA, central macular thickness (CMT) and need for additional laser therapy. Median VA results were better for 0.3mg (65 letters), as compared with sham (60 letters) ($p=0.04$) and 34% of patients receiving 0.3mg gained $\geq 10$ letters vs. 10% for sham. Mean CMT decreased by 68μm with 0.3mg, vs. 4μm increase with sham. Laser treatment was deemed necessary in fewer cases treated with pegaptanib (25%) than with sham (48%). The safety profile was good with only one case of endophthalmitis in 652 injections and was not associated with severe visual loss.

Six years later the results of a phase 2/3, randomized, 2-year trial of pegaptanib for the treatment of DME were released [25]. 260 patients were evaluated during the first year and 207 patients during the second year. VA gain was ≥ 10 letters in 37% of the patients treated with pegaptanib vs. 20% of those treated with sham at week 54. At week 102, the average VA gain in the pegaptanib group was 6.1 letters vs. 1.3 letters for sham, and 25% of the treated eyes had required laser treatment by the end of the second year vs. 45% in the sham group. Similarly, pegaptanib-treated patients did better in the National Eye Institute-Visual Functioning Questionnaire (NEI-VFQ) than sham. Pegaptanib safety was good and the frequency of discontinuations, adverse events, treatment-related adverse events, and serious adverse events was similar in both groups. One of the main advantages of treatment with pegaptanib is its high specificity for the ocular isoform of VEGF and its excellent safety profile. However, and even though results from this trials were better than the conventional outcome for laser treatment, intravitreal pegaptanib has not been considered a first line treatment for DME. A recent PubMed search using the key words *pegaptanib* and *DME* produced only 30 references, most of them from revisions on the subject. Our group reported on one eye with DME treated by intravitreal pegaptanib that presented a detachment of the posterior hyaloid that might have, at least in part, helped in the resolution of DME, even though VA remained unchanged [26]. Among the few original papers on the use of pegaptanib we may mention a small retrospective series by Querques et al. on the outcomes of primary intravitreal pegaptanib in patients with DME. These authors compared the results of 13 eyes treated primarily with pegaptanib with eyes treated with pegaptanib associated with macular laser photocoagulation and eyes treated with primary macular laser photocoagulation. Eyes treated with pegaptanib as monotherapy showed significant VA improvement and reduction in macular thickness ($p=0.0014$ and $p=0.0001$) that were not observed in the laser monotherapy and combined treatment groups [27].

In summary, pegaptanib has been found to be more effective than laser treatment as monotherapy for DME involving the center of the macula. Even though its efficacy might be slightly worse than other non-selective VEGF blockers, the number of patients with significant VA gain after treatment are similar to those treated with non-selective VEGF blockers, while showing a better ocular and systemic safety profile [28].

Pfizer Pharmaceuticals is no longer pursuing further studies for pegaptanib in DME.

## RANIBIZUMAB (LUCENTIS®, GENENTECH, NOVARTIS)

Ranibizumab (Lucentis Novartis Pharma AG, Basel, Switzerland and Genentech Inc., South San Francisco, CA, US) is a fully humanized monoclonal antibody fragment that binds to multiple variants of VEGFA. Ranibizumab was approved by the Food and Drug Administration (FDA) and the European Medicines Agency (EMEA) for the treatment of visual impairment due to DME, based on evidence from two pivotal trials, RESOLVE and RESTORE. Presently, ranibizumab gathers the most robust evidence based on prospective clinical trials treating patients with DME.

Chun et al. performed a single-center, open-label, dose-escalating pilot study on 10 eyes from 10 patients with VA between 60 and 20 letters in order to evaluate the biologic activity of intravitreal ranibizumab (IVR) in patients with center-involving clinically significant DME [29]. They performed three IVR (0.3mg or 0.5mg) on day 0, month 1, and month 2, and followed by observation until month 24 in order to evaluate frequency and severity of ocular and systemic adverse events, as well as VA and retinal thickness changes by OCT. IVR was well tolerated and no systemic adverse events were reported. At month 3, 4 of 10 patients gained ≥15 letters, and 5 of 10 gained ≥10 letters, with a mean decrease in CMT of 45.3±196.3μm for the 0.3mg group and 197.8±85.9μm for the 0.5mg group. In the RESOLVE trial three consecutive monthly IVR (0.3 or 0.5mg) were administered and followed by *pro re nata* (PRN) regimen with predefined retreatment criteria. Dose doubling and rescue laser were permitted at investigator discretion. The primary efficacy outcome was the mean average VA change over 12 months, from baseline. The mean average change in VA with ranibizumab was superior to that of the sham control group (10.3 letters with a mean of 10 injections vs. a loss of 1.4 letters in the sham group). More patients receiving IVR gained ≥15 letters compared with patients receiving sham injections.

Dose doubling was more frequent in the sham arm (92%) than in the ranibizumab arm (69%), and a higher proportion of patients in the sham arm received rescue laser therapy (33%) compared with ranibizumab (5%) [30].

Following these good results, the READ 2 study compared IVR with focal/grid laser or a combination of both in eyes with DME [31]. 126 patients with DME were randomized 1:1:1 to receive 0.5mg of IVR at baseline and months 1, 3, and 5, focal/grid laser photocoagulation at baseline and month 3 (if needed) or a combination of both at baseline and month 3. At month 6, the mean gain in VA was significantly greater in eyes treated with IVR (+7.24 letters, $p=0.01$, analysis of variance) compared with the laser group (-0.43 letters). There were no statistically significant difference between the group treated by combined therapy (+3.80 letters) and either of the monotherapy groups. Eight of 37 eyes treated by IVR monotherapy gained ≥ 3 lines by month 6 vs. 0 of 38 of the eyes treated by laser monotherapy ($p=0.002$, Fisher exact test) and 3 of 40 with combined therapy. Foveal thickness decreased by 50%, 33%, and 45% respectively. After month 6, all subjects could be treated with IVR if retreatment criteria were met. The mean number of injections after month 6 was 5.3, 4.4, and 2.9 respectively, for a mean improvement in VA of 7.7, 5.1, and 6.8 letters at month 24. The percentage of patients who gained ≥ 3 lines was 24, 18 and 26 respectively at month 24. Mean CMT at month 24 was 340µm, 286µm, and 258µm respectively, showing an anatomical benefit of combined therapy.

The RESTORE trial was a much larger randomized, double-masked, laser-controlled phase III study aimed at demonstrating the superiority of IVR 0.5mg monotherapy or combined with laser over laser alone [32]. 345 patients with type 1 or 2 DM and DME were randomized to IVR + sham laser, ranibizumab + laser, or sham injections + laser. Ranibizumab/sham was given for 3 months followed by PRN regime while laser/sham laser was given at baseline followed by PRN. The results proved that IVR as monotherapy and combined treatment was superior to laser monotherapy in terms of VA gain (+6.1 and +5.9 vs.+0.8; $p<0.0001$). At month 12 VA gain was ≥15 letters and letter score was ≥73 with IVR monotherapy (22.6% and 53%, respectively) and combined therapy (22.9% and 44.9%) vs. laser monotherapy (8.2% and 23.6%). Similarly, mean CMT was significantly reduced from baseline with IVR (-118.7µm) and combined therapy (-128.3µm) vs. laser (-61.3µm; both $p<0.001$). The NEI VFQ-25 questionnaire also showed improved quality of life among IVR treated eyes vs. laser. The mean number of injections performed over 12 months was 7 ranibizumab/sham injections. The ocular and systemic safety profile was excellent with no case of endophthalmitis and only 2 cases of increased intraocular pressure (IOP) among the IVR treated eyes, and without an increased risk of cardiovascular or cerebrovascular events.

The RIDE and RISE trials assessed the effects of IVR in DME controlled with sham injections on 759 eyes with DME during 3 years [33]. Patients were randomized to monthly 0.5mg or 0.3mg IVR or sham injections during two years, and then sham patients were eligible to cross over to monthly 0.5mg IVR. Macular laser was permitted to all patients from month 3 onwards and panretinal laser as necessary. VA outcomes at month 24 in IVR treated groups were consistent through month 36. As in the previous studies, VA gain was much higher among the IVR treated eyes: the proportions of patients who gained ≥15 letters from baseline in the sham (crossed over to 0.5mg), 0.3mg, and 0.5mg IVR groups were 19%, 37%, and 40%, respectively in the RIDE study and 22%, 51%, and 42%, respectively, in the RISE study. VA gains after crossover to 1 year of treatment with IVR in the sham/ 0.5mg group were lower compared with the IVR patients after 1 year of treatment (2.8 vs. 10.6 and 11.1 letters). The safety profile was good with an incidence of 0.06% endophthalmitis per injection. However, the incidence of serious cardiovascular adverse events was 20% and 17% in patients who received 0.5mg and 0.3mg IVR, respectively.

The Diabetic Retinopathy Clinical Research Network (DRCR.net) Protocol I Study was an independent, randomized, phase III trial performed on 854 eyes with central macular thickening due to DME. Patients were treated by IVR plus either prompt (within 3-10 days of IVR) or deferred (≥24 weeks after IVR) combined treatment (TA plus laser) or laser monotherapy. IVR was performed at baseline and every 4 weeks until week 12. Afterwards, retreatment was performed at investigator discretion guided by predefined VA and OCT. Follow-up was meant to be 5 years. Mean VA change from baseline to year 1 was significantly better with IVR combined with either type of laser monotherapy treatment. A mean improvement of 9 letters was achieved with a median of 8 and 9 IVR in the prompt and deferred laser groups, respectively. VA gain at year 1 was sustained during year 2, with a median of only two and three IVR in the ranibizumab plus prompt and deferred laser groups, respectively.

One of the main drawbacks of IVR is the high cost. Therefore, it has been associated with laser treatment in order to reduce the number of injections while maintaining VA gain. Dewan et al. performed a cost-effectiveness analysis of the treatment of diabetic macular edema (DME) with IVR plus prompt (R+pL) or deferred laser (R+dL) vs. TA plus prompt laser (TA+L) [34], using the data from reports of the DRCR.net Protocol I. According to their results, effectiveness through 2 years for sham plus laser (S+L), R+pL or R+dL, and TA+L was predicted to be 3.46, 7.07, 8.63, and 2.40 letters, respectively. The ICER values in terms of dollars per VA letter were \$393 (S+L vs. TA+L), \$5943 (R+pL vs. S+L), and \$20 (R+dL vs. R+pL). For pseudophakics, the ICER value for comparison TA with laser vs. IVR with deferred laser was \$14 690 per letter gained. IVR with deferred laser provided an additional 6 letters correct compared with TA with laser at an additional cost of \$19 216 over 2 years, suggesting that if the gain in VA was maintained in subsequent years, the treatment of phakic patients with DME using IVR might meet accepted standards of cost-effectiveness, whereas first-line treatment with TA seemed to be the most cost-effective option in pseudophakic patients.

Stein et al. tried to determine the most cost-effective treatment option for patients with recently diagnosed clinically significant DME, among focal laser photocoagulation alone (L), focal laser plus IVR (L+R), focal laser plus intravitreal bevacizumab (L+B), or focal laser plus intravitreal TA (L+TA) injections [35]. They compared the incremental cost-effectiveness of treating patients with newly diagnosed clinically significant DME using L, L+R, L+B, or L+TA. Data were obtained from the DRCR.net randomized controlled trial, the Medicare fee schedule, and the medical literature. According to their results, the incremental cost-effectiveness of L+R and L+B compared with laser monotherapy was \$89 903/QALY and \$11 138/QALY, respectively. The authors concluded that bevacizumab therapy conferred the greatest value among the different treatment options for clinically significant DME.

Ranibizumab has also been compared with intravitreal TA. Elman et al. reported on a 2 year randomized study that compared IVR 0.5mg vs. 4mg TA combined with focal/grid laser vs. focal/grid laser alone for treatment of DME performed on 854 eyes of 691 patients with VA between 75 and 25 letters and central macular edema [36]. At two years the mean VA gain was 3.7 in patients on IVR + prompt laser group (compared with the sham + prompt laser Group), 5.8 letters in the IVR + deferred laser group and 1.5 letters lost in the TA + prompt laser group. Similarly, by the end of the second year the percentages of eyes with CMT ≥250μm were 59% in the sham + prompt laser group, 43% in the IVR + prompt laser group, 42% in the IVR + deferred laser group, and 52% in the TA + prompt laser group. Systemic safety was good, with no systemic events attributable to study treatments. Three eyes in 375 patients treated by IVR had injection-related endophthalmitis, and elevated IOP and cataract surgery were more frequent in the TA + prompt laser group.

Ollendorf assessed the comparative effectiveness of anti-VEGF therapy in the treatment of DME, based on a literature search concerning treatment of DME with aflibercept, bevacizumab, pegaptanib, or ranibizumab between

2000 and 2012, compared to laser photocoagulation, sham injection, or TA [37]. Effectiveness was based on VA gain. The authors evaluated 15 randomized controlled trials and eight observational studies. All agents permitted VA gain ranging 4-9 letters. However, meta-analyses showed no statistically significant differences between agents in terms of VA change or the ratio of patients gaining ≥10 letters. Similar results were obtained comparing the potential harms of anti-VEGFs, including ocular events, heart infarct, stroke, and other cardiovascular events, as well as death, concluding that evidence is insufficient to distinguish the performance of any single anti-VEGF agent over others.

Since VEGF is expressed as a response to ischemia, it might be expected that anti-VEGF drugs might increase the effects of retinal ischemia. Campochiaro evaluated the effects of VEGF suppression by monthly IVR on posterior retinal non-perfusion (RNP) in patients with DME [38], by a retrospective analysis of prospectively collected data from two randomized, sham injection-controlled, double-masked, multicenter clinical trials. An independent reading center measured the area of RNP on FA obtained in the phase 3 RISE and RIDE trials in 666 patients with DME. The percentage of patients with no posterior RNP decreased in the sham group between baseline and month 24, but remained relatively stable in the two ranibizumab groups. Patients from the sham group were crossed over to receive monthly IVR 0.5mg after month 24, and the differences between the sham and IVR groups were reduced. Initiation of IVR in the sham group at month 24 was followed by reduction in the percentage of patients with an increase in posterior RNP from baseline at months 30 and 36, whereas the two IVR groups continued their gradual rise. The authors concluded that high VEGF levels contribute to progression of retinal non-perfusion in patients with DME, suggesting that high levels of VEGF can cause closure of retinal vessels, and monthly IVR can slow down, but not completely prevent, retinal capillary closure in patients with DME. IVR has been shown to be superior to macular laser photocoagulation and intraocular TA injections for improving visual acuity and drying the macula. Most experts now consider intravitreal anti-VEGF therapy to be standard-of-care for DME involving the fovea [39].

## Bevacizumab (Avastin®, Roche, Genentech)

Bevacizumab is an antiangiogenic drug licensed as an antineoplastic agent that derives from a recombinant humanized monoclonal IgG1 antibody and inhibits VEGF. Bevacizumab is used clinically as an off-label treatment in the treatment of exudative AMD and myopic choroidal neovascularization, as well as DME and macular edema secondary to retinal vein occlusion.

The DRCR.net performed a phase II trial including 121 eyes with DME over a 12-week period to assess the effect of intravitreal bevacizumab (IVB) [40]. Sixty-nine percent of the included eyes were refractory to previous treatment. The eyes were randomized into five groups to be treated by (I) focal laser, (II) two injections of 1.25mg IVB at 0 and 6weeks, (III) two injections of 2.5mg IVB at 0 and 6 weeks, (IV) injection of 1.25mg IVB at baseline and sham injection at 6 weeks or (V) injection of 1.25mg IVB at baseline and 6 weeks with photocoagulation at 3 weeks. Groups II and III had a significant VA gain over the laser monotherapy group (I) throughout the 12 weeks that was associated with greater improvement in CMT at the 3-week visit. No differences were observed between the two different doses of bevacizumab (1.25mg vs. 2.5mg), and the single injection group was not superior to the laser group. Combined treatment showed results similar to laser-only treatment. Eyes that received primary treatment had greater improvement than the refractory ones.

A randomized clinical trial compared IVB injection alone or combined with IVT vs. macular laser photocoagulation as a primary treatment for DME. (41) A total of 150 eyes from 129 patients were randomly assigned to the following groups: (I) 1.25mg IVB, (II) 1.25mg IVB and 2mg IVT, and (III) macular laser. The IVB group showed significantly higher VA gain after six months that was not sustained after 24 months. Mean VA was significantly better in the IVB group compared to baseline after 6 months.

The Pan-American Collaborative Retina Study Group (PACORES) examined IVB as the primary treatment for diffuse DME in a retrospective, multicenter, interventional, comparative case series on 139 eyes with diffuse DME treated with at least one off-label IVB of either 1.25 or 2.5mg [42]. The dose received at baseline was the same dose delivered throughout the study. Follow-up considered VA and OCT at baseline and 1, 3, 6, 12, and 24 months. The reinjection criterion was recurrence of diffuse DME. No significant differences were observed between the 1.25mg and 2.5mg doses. Mean VA and CMT improved at 1 month and were sustainable all along the 24 months. By month 24, 52% of the eyes improved by ≥2 ETDRS lines, 45% remained stable, and 4% decreased by ≥2 lines. The mean number of injections per eye was 5.8 (ranging 1-15).

The bevacizumab or laser therapy study (BOLT) was a prospective, randomized, masked, single-center study that compared IVB to macular laser photocoagulation in persistent DME after at least one macular laser treatment [43]. Eighty eyes were randomized to IVB every 6 weeks (with a minimum of 3 and a maximum of 9 injections), or laser treatment every 4 months (with a minimum of 1 and a maximum of 4). Mean VA after 1 year increased in the IVB group and declined in the laser group. Macular thickness was lower in the bevacizumab group as well. The mean number of IVB was 9 vs. 3 laser treatments during the first year. The 2-year report presented similar results to those of the first year report, with a mean VA of 65 letters in the IVB group vs. 55 letters in the laser group and a mean gain of 8.6 letters vs. 0.5 letters respectively [44]. CMT decreased significantly in both groups at 2-year follow-up and the mean number of treatments was 13 IVB vs. 4 laser interventions, supporting the longer-term use of IVB for the treatment of DME [45].

The Canadian Agency for Drugs and Technologies in Health performed a systematic review of IVB for the treatment of DME [46], based on randomized controlled trials (open-label, single-masked, or double-masked) comparing IVB with placebo/sham or other treatments in patients with DME. The authors evaluated ten trials: one of IVB vs. sham injections [47]; five vs. laser therapy [41, 43, 48-50]; and four vs. intravitreal TA [51-54]. Three studies included primarily patients with type 2 DM. No trials directly compared IVB with IVR in patients with DME. Mortality and serious adverse events (SAEs) did not differ, with two deaths out of 369 eyes treated with IVB compared with five deaths out of 314 eyes treated with comparators (p=0.20), and 29/369 SAEs on IVB vs. 20/314 for comparators (p=0.45).

Ahmadieh et al. compared IVB with sham treatment in 78 patients with DME refractory to laser therapy, during 6 months [47]. VA gain was not seen with IVB at week six, but differed significantly from sham at weeks 12 to 24, with a VA gain of approximately 11 ETDRS letters with IVB vs. sham, and decreased CMT vs. sham at six and 24 weeks, though results were not significant at 12 and 18 weeks. Regarding safety, eight eyes presented mild anterior chamber reactions and one eye progressed to fibrous proliferation, though no patient was withdrawn from the trial due to adverse events.

Five trials compared IVB to laser photocoagulation in a total of 396 eyes. Three of them assessed VA at six weeks and found that IVB provided a significant mean improvement of 9 ETDRS letters vs. laser. The difference was not statistically significant at weeks 12, 16, or 24 [41, 48, 49]. Michaelides et al. reported VA at 12 months with a median gain of eight letters in the IVB group vs. a median loss of 0.5 letters in the laser group (p=0.0002) [43]. In these five trials, four eyes had increased IOP and one eye developed endophthalmitis in the IVB group vs. none in the laser group. A total number of 48/223 adverse events were reported in the IVB group vs. 20/173 (12%) in the laser group. Mean change in CMT did not differ significantly between IVB and laser at week six and at week 24, laser performed better than IVB, with a mean difference of 37.86μm (p=0.002).

Four trials compared IVB with TA (n = 209 eyes in total). Shahin and El-Lakkany [54] (n = 48 eyes) reported on 58% of the eyes on TA gaining ≥ two ETDRS lines vs. none on IVB. They also reported deterioration in ≥ 1 ETDRS line in three IVB eyes and zero in TA eyes. However this trial had inadequate masking, resulting in a high risk of bias.

Paccola et al., and Marey and Ellakwa reported that VA was significantly better on TA than IVB at weeks 6, 12, and 24 [52, 53], with a mean difference of eight, six, and five ETDRS letters, respectively, though as in the previous case, both trials had either inadequate allocation concealment and masking, or inadequate reporting on methods. Increased IOP occurred in 8/50 (16%) eyes on TA vs. zero on IVB in two trials [51, 54].

Ozturk et al. performed a direct comparison of IVB and IVR on visual function and CMT in patients with DME [55]. The authors revised the data of diabetic patients who received 1 injection of IVB and IVR with at least 6-month interval, and recorded VA and CMT before and after the injections. They included 29 eyes of 29 patients with a median VA and CMT of 59 ETDRS letters and 411μm respectively before the IVB. Four to six weeks after the injection, median VA increased to 61.5 ETDRS letters and the median CMT decreased to 373μm (p=0.029 and p=0.011, respectively). After a mean 9.54±2.64 months interval IVR treatment was performed, that increased the median VA from 53 to 66 letters and decreased the median CMT from 428 to 279μm (p<0.001 and p<0.001, respectively). The median change in VA was 4.5 ETDRS letters in the IVB group and 6 letters in the IVR group (p=0.58), whereas the median changes in CMT were 41 and 100μm after IVB and IVR, respectively (p=0.005).

We have performed a retrospective study on 44 patients with DME treated by IVB that presented a baseline VA of 58.1±11.9 ETDRS letters, with an average CMT of 536±12μm. Patients′ mean age was 70 ± 7 years and they had been diabetic during an average of 14 ± 8 years. The mean number of IVB performed during the first year was 4.1±1.7, and by the end of the first year VA was 60.7±13.9 letters. The results are shown in Table 1. Our results suggest a moderate VA gain followed by stabilization after IVB that was associated with a limited improvement in retinal thickness. However, it should be noted that the number of IVB was markedly lower than what is usually reported in the published series.

In a previous, unpublished study performed by our group, two patients with bilateral diffuse DME were treated by monthly IVR in the left eye (LE). VA and CMT determinations were monthly performed by certified personnel. Three consecutive monthly injections were given, and further re injections were performed whenever VA loss or CMT increase were detected.

Following decreased CMT and improved VA in the treated eye (LE), and CMT and VA deterioration in the fellow, untreated eye (right eye, RE), treatment was discussed with the patients.

**Table 1. Baseline and post treatment visual acuity and central macular thickness after intravitreal bevacizumab**

| | VA (ETDRS letters) | CMT (µm) | # IVB |
|---|---|---|---|
| **Baseline** | **58.1±11.9** | **536±12** | |
| **12 months** | **60.7±13.9** | **400±126** | **4.1±1.7** |
| **24 months** | **54.8±14.8** | **355±161** | **1.8±1.9** |
| **36 months** | **60±18** | **468±317** | **1.3±1.5** |
| **48 months** | **55±28** | **312±265** | **2.5±3.5** |

Due to the high cost of the treatment, monthly IVB was performed in the RE. The results are shown in Figures 5-7. Two to four months after the last IVR in the LE, CMT and VA worsened, forcing repeated IVR. However, the response to IVB was less noticeable in terms of CMT and almost negligible in terms of VA. Rescue therapy on the RE was tried using intravitreal TA, achieving an effective reduction of CMT as well as a moderate improvement in VA. The different efficacy of bevacizumab and ranibizumab may be related to the differences in pharmacokinetics between both drugs that will permit a smaller molecule such as ranibizumab to reach deeper into the retina [56].

## Aflibercept (Eylea®, Bayer, Regeneron Pharmaceuticals)

Aflibercept (EYLEA®-Regeneron Pharmaceuticals, Inc., Tarrytown, New York, NY, and Bayer Healthcare Pharmaceuticals, Berlin, Germany), also known as VEGF Trap-Eye is a new 115-kDa anti-VEGF agent. It is a fusion protein developed with the "trap technology". The extracellular binding domains of VEGF receptors (VEGFR) -1 and -2 are combined to the Fc segment of human immunoglobulin-G1. As occurs with ranibizumab and bevacizumab, aflibercept binds to all isomers of the VEGFA family, plus VEGFB and PlGF, what might increase its efficacy. Aflibercept binds firmly to the target and inhibits binding and activation of the VEGF receptors. The affinity of aflibercept to VEGFA as occurs with the union between efector and receptor is much higher than that of monoclonal anti-VEGF antibodies (5 pM kD vs.1 pM kD), and binds to VEGF 140 times more powerfully than ranibizumab, creating a one-month intravitreal binding activity that exceeds both ranibizumab and bevacizumab.

According to a predictive mathematical model by Stewart et al. [57], aflibercept is active in the eye for 10 to 12 weeks after a single intravitreal injection, and the binding activity of 2mg aflibercept at 83 days is estimated to be comparable to that of 0.5mg ranibizumab at 30 days. The half-life in the human eye has not yet been identified but in animals it is considered to be about 5 days.

In 2009, a phase-I study was performed to assess the safety, tolerability and bioactivity of a single 4mg injection of aflibercept in DME over a period of 6 weeks [58]. The biological activity was measured by changes in VA and in the retinal thickness assessed by OCT.

According to this trial, a single intravitreal injection of 4mg of aflibercept was well tolerated, improving VA and reducing CMT. The median VA gain was 9 letters after 4 weeks and 3 letters after 6 weeks. Based on the results of the phase I study, a 52 week, multicenter, randomized, double-masked, active-controlled phase II clinical trial was conducted, in order to assess the safety and efficacy of intravitreal aflibercept vs. focal/grid laser photocoagulation in patients with DME. This trial enrolled 221 subjects with center-involved DME and VA between 70 and 25 letters that were randomized into 5 groups: 0.5mg aflibercept every 4 weeks (0.5q4), 2.0mg every 4 weeks (2q4), 2.0mg monthly for 3 months and then every 8 weeks (2q8), 2.0mg monthly for 3 months and then as needed (2 PRN), and macular laser treatment. All aflibercept groups received sham laser and all laser patients received sham injection. The primary endpoint was the mean change in VA; and the change in CMT and the number of patients gaining ≥ 15 letters at week 24 were secondary outcomes. Improvement in mean change of VA from 8.5 to 11.4 letters was observed in aflibercept groups vs. 2.5 letters in the laser group at week 24. CMT decreased more in the aflibercept groups compared to the laser group. No significant differences were seen between the aflibercept groups, supporting the promising idea of a treatment regimen of every 8 weeks. The one-year results showed an average gain ranging from 9.7 to 13.1 letters in the aflibercept groups vs. a loss of 1.3 letters in the laser group [59].

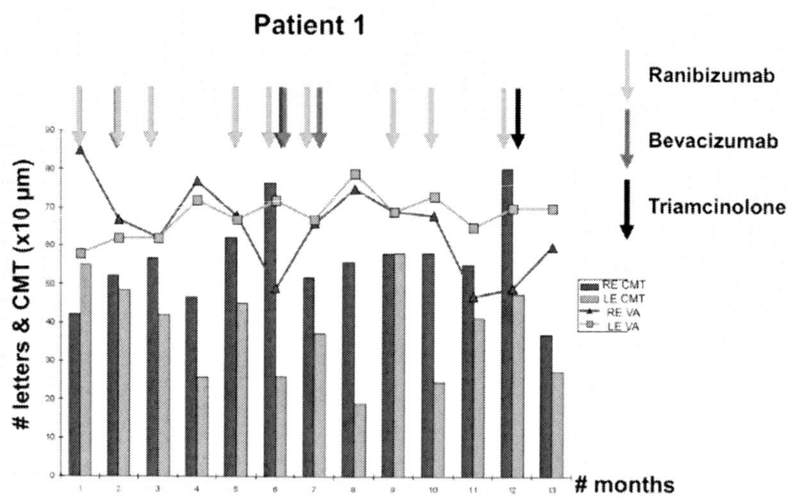


Figure 5. Flow chart of intravitreal injections of ranibizumab (blue) (in the left eye, LE) and bevacizumab (red) and triamcinolone (black) (in the right eye, RE) in patient #1. The lines show changes in visual acuity (VA) for the LE (blue) and RE (red) and the bars show changes in macular thickness (CMT) for the LE (blue) and RE (red).

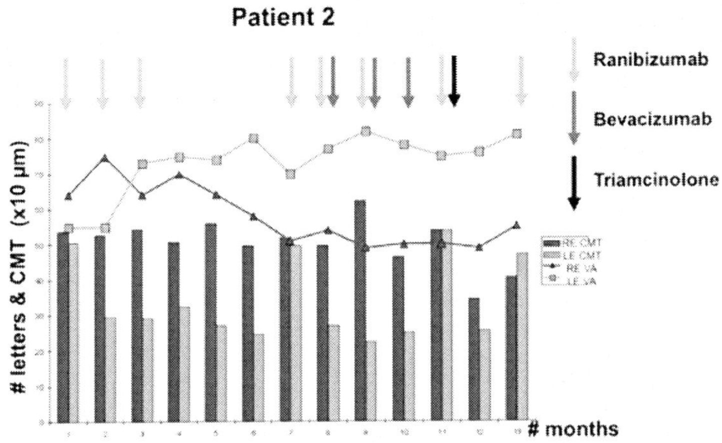


Figure 6. Flow chart of intravitreal injections of ranibizumab (blue) (in the left eye, LE) and bevacizumab (red) and triamcinolone (black) (in the right eye, RE) in patient #2. The lines show changes in visual acuity (VA) for the LE (blue) and RE (red) and the bars show changes in macular thickness (CMT) for the LE (blue) and RE (red).

Two phase III trials have been recently reported. VIVID-DME (NCT01331681) and VISTA-DME (NCT01363440) are randomized, double-masked, active controlled trials that investigate the efficacy and safety of repeated doses of intravitreal aflibercept in 865 patients with DME. Patients were randomized (1:1:1) to receive either 2.0mg aflibercept every 4 weeks (2q4) or 2.0mg aflibercept every 8 weeks after 5 initial monthly doses (2q8) or laser photocoagulation. After the first year, the primary results showed the superiority of aflibercept over laser treatment. Mean VA gain in the VIVID-DME study was 10.7 letters in the 2q8 group and 10.5 in the 2q4 vs. 1.2 in the laser group.

The VISTA-DME showed a similar VA gain of 10.7 letters in the 2q8, 12.5 in the 2q4, and 0.2 in the laser group. Secondary outcomes, showed a significant superiority of aflibercept over laser treatment in terms of reduction of macular thickness, proportion of patients gaining ≥15 letters and improvement of Diabetic Retinopathy Severity Score. The aflibercept 2q8 group performed similarly as the aflibercept 2q4 group.

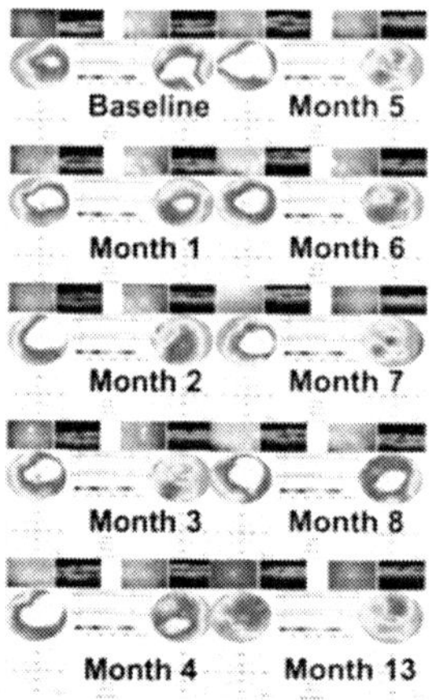


Figure 7. OCT changes in macular thickness following ranibizumab, bevacizumab and triamcinolone as shown for patient #1. Notice the macular thickness decrease in the left eye following the intravitreal injections of ranibizumab as macular thickness increases in the right, untreated eye.

# TREATMENT PROTOCOLS

## Spanish Vitreo Retina Society

The Spanish Vitreo Retina Society recommends the following algorithms for the management of DME (Tables 2 and 3) [60].

### Table 2. Guidelines for the management of diabetic macular edema

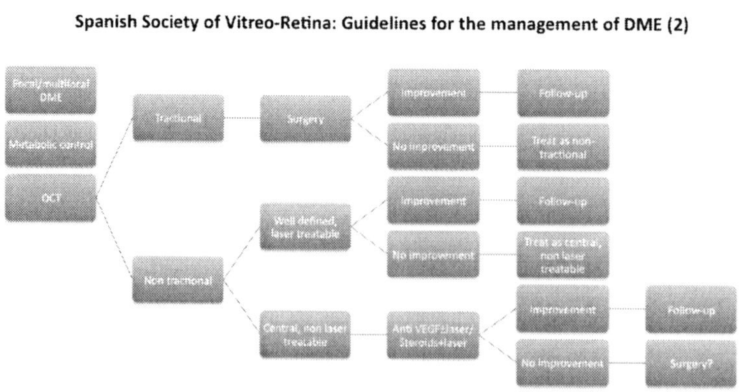

**Table 3. Guidelines for the management of diabetic macular edema**

**Spanish Society of Vitreo-Retina: Guidelines for the management of DME (2)**

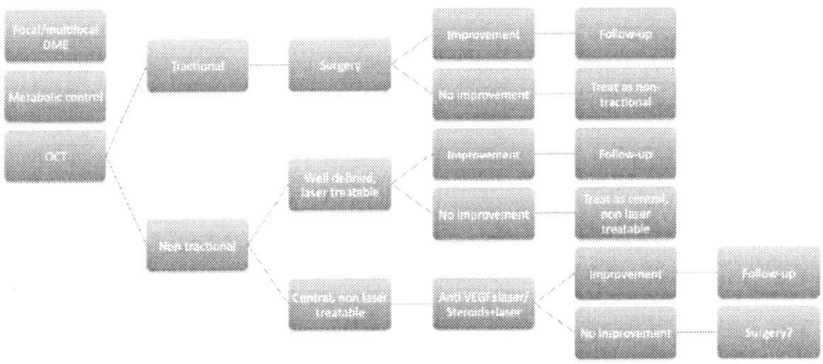


**Table 4. Guidelines for the management of diabetic macular edema**

**The Royal College of Ophthalmologists: Diabetic Retinopathy Guidelines**

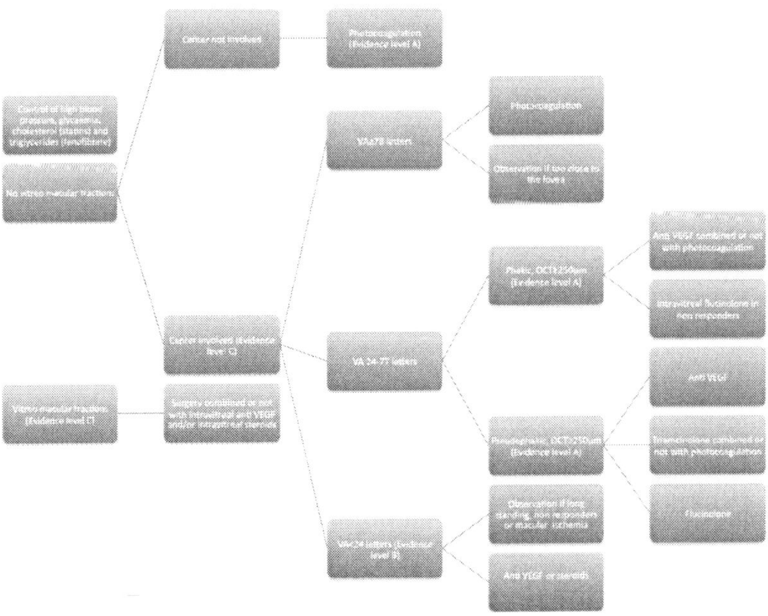


The Royal College of Ophthalmologists recommends the algorithm adapted in Table 4 [61].

It is recommended that intravitreal anti-VEGF treatment should be performed monthly during a loading phase of 4-6 months followed by PRN treatment until the macula is dry or no further improvement is expected. Monthly follow-up is suggested during at least 2 years, and afterwards controls should be performed every 12 to 16 weeks.

## CONCLUSION

DME is an important cause of vision impairment. Recent studies have revealed significantly positive visual and anatomical results regarding the use of anti-VEGF for the treatment of DME. Anti-VEGF therapy has assumed an important role in the management of DME, either as a monotherapy or as adjuvant to photocoagulation. Safety issues concerning intravitreal injection of anti-VEGF are still a concern though they are well known from AMD studies in elderly patients. Serious ocular adverse events are infrequent and include traumatic cataract, endophthalmitis, uveitis, and retinal detachment. Systemic adverse events include death, myocardial infarction, arterial hypertension and stroke. The small number of relevant trials limits comparisons between different anti-VEGF drugs. Presently ranibizumab is the only approved anti-VEGF for DME, though the markedly lower cost of bevacizumab and the potential of aflibercept to decrease treatment burden and associated cost are to be considered.

## REFERENCES

[1] Mitchell, P., Foran, S. *Guidelines for the Management of Diabetic Retinopathy*. In: (NHMRC) TNHaMRC, editor. Canberra, Australia: Australian Diabetes Society for the Department of Health and Aging; 2008.

[2] Photocoagulation for diabetic macular edema. Early Treatment Diabetic Retinopathy Study report number 1. Early Treatment Diabetic Retinopathy Study research group. *Arch. Ophthalmol*. 1985 Dec.;103 (12):1796-806.

[3] Sivaprasad, S., Dorin, G. Subthreshold diode laser micropulse photocoagulation for the treatment of diabetic macular edema. *Expert Rev. Med. Devices*. 2012 Mar.;9(2):189-97.

[4] Shimura, M., Yasuda, K., Nakazawa, T., Ota, S., Tamai, M. Effective treatment of diffuse diabetic macular edema by temporal grid pattern photocoagulation. *Ophthalmic Surg. Lasers Imaging*. 2004 Jul.-Aug.;35 (4):270-80.

[5] Olk, R. J., Akduman, L. Minimal intensity diode laser (810 nanometer) photocoagulation (MIP) for diffuse diabetic macular edema (DDME). *Semin. Ophthalmol.* 2001 Mar.;16(1):25-30.

[6] Tunc, M., Onder, H. I., Kaya, M. Posterior sub-Tenon's capsule triamcinolone injection combined with focal laser photocoagulation for diabetic macular edema. *Ophthalmology*. 2005 Jun.;112(6):1086-91.

[7] Martidis, A., Duker, J. S., Greenberg, P. B., Rogers, A. H., Puliafito, C. A., Reichel, E., et al. Intravitreal triamcinolone for refractory diabetic macular edema. *Ophthalmology*. 2002 May;109(5):920-7.

[8] Jonas, J. B., Kreissig, I., Sofker, A., Degenring, R. F. Intravitreal injection of triamcinolone for diffuse diabetic macular edema. *Arch. Ophthalmol.* 2003 Jan.;121(1):57-61.

[9] Jonas, J. B., Degenring, R., Kreissig, I., Akkoyun, I. Safety of intravitreal high-dose reinjections of triamcinolone acetonide. *Am. J. Ophthalmol.* 2004 Dec.;138(6):1054-5.

[10] Montero, J. A., Ruiz-Moreno, J. M. Intravitreal inserts of steroids to treat diabetic macular edema. *Curr. Diabetes Rev*. 2009 Feb.;5(1):26-32.

[11] Michaelson, I. C. Vascular morphogenesis in the retina of the cat. *J. Anat.* 1948 Jul.;82(3):167-74.

[12] Senger, D. R., Connolly, D. T., Van de Water, L., Feder, J., Dvorak, H. F. Purification and NH2-terminal amino acid sequence of guinea pig tumor-secreted vascular permeability factor. *Cancer Res.* 1990 Mar. 15; 50(6):1774-8.

[13] Ferrara, N., Henzel, W. J. Pituitary follicular cells secrete a novel heparin-binding growth factor specific for vascular endothelial cells. *Biochem. Biophys. Res. Commun.* 1989 Jun. 15;161(2):851-8.

[14] Gerber, H. P., McMurtrey, A., Kowalski, J., Yan, M., Keyt, B. A., Dixit, V., et al. Vascular endothelial growth factor regulates endothelial cell survival through the phosphatidylinositol 3'-kinase/Akt signal transduction pathway. Requirement for Flk-1/KDR activation. *J. Biol. Chem.* 1998 Nov. 13;273(46):30336-43.

[15] Ferrara, N. Vascular endothelial growth factor: basic science and clinical progress. *Endocr. Rev*. 2004 Aug.;25(4):581-611.

[16] Jain, R. K. Normalization of tumor vasculature: an emerging concept in antiangiogenic therapy. *Science*. 2005 Jan. 7;307(5706):58-62.

[17] Aiello, L. P., Avery, R. L., Arrigg, P. G., Keyt, B. A., Jampel, H. D., Shah, S. T., et al. Vascular endothelial growth factor in ocular fluid of patients with diabetic retinopathy and other retinal disorders. *N. Engl. J. Med.* 1994 Dec. 1;331(22):1480-7.

[18] Wang, K., Wang, Y., Gao, L., Li, X., Li, M., Guo, J. Dexamethasone inhibits leukocyte accumulation and vascular permeability in retina of streptozotocin-induced diabetic rats via reducing vascular endothelial growth factor and intercellular adhesion molecule-1 expression. *Biol. Pharm. Bull.* 2008 Aug.;31(8):1541-6.

[19] Funatsu, H., Yamashita, H., Ikeda, T., Mimura, T., Eguchi, S., Hori, S. Vitreous levels of interleukin-6 and vascular endothelial growth factor are related to diabetic macular edema. *Ophthalmology*. 2003 Sep.; 110 (9):1690-6.

[20] Itakura, H., Kishi, S., Kotajima, N., Murakami, M. Persistent secretion of vascular endothelial growth factor into the vitreous cavity in proliferative diabetic retinopathy after vitrectomy. *Ophthalmology*. 2004 Oct.;111(10):1880-4.

[21] Zehetner, C., Kirchmair, R., Huber, S., Kralinger, M. T., Kieselbach, G. F. Plasma levels of vascular endothelial growth factor before and after intravitreal injection of bevacizumab, ranibizumab and pegaptanib in patients with age-related macular degeneration, and in patients with diabetic macular oedema. *Br. J. Ophthalmol.* 2013 Apr.;97(4):454-9.

[22] Gragoudas, E. S., Adamis, A. P., Cunningham, E. T., Jr., Feinsod, M., Guyer, D. R. Pegaptanib for neovascular age-related macular degeneration. *N. Engl. J. Med.* 2004 Dec. 30;351(27):2805-16.

[23] Rosenfeld, P. J., Brown, D. M., Heier, J. S., Boyer, D. S., Kaiser, P. K., Chung, C. Y., et al. Ranibizumab for neovascular age-related macular degeneration. *N. Engl. J. Med.* 2006 Oct. 5;355(14):1419-31.

[24] Cunningham, E. T., Jr., Adamis, A. P., Altaweel, M., Aiello, L. P., Bressler, N. M., D'Amico, D. J., et al. A phase II randomized double-masked trial of pegaptanib, an anti-vascular endothelial growth factor aptamer, for diabetic macular edema. *Ophthalmology*. 2005 Oct.; 112 (10):1747-57.

[25] Sultan, M. B., Zhou, D., Loftus, J., Dombi, T., Ice, K. S. A phase 2/3, multicenter, randomized, double-masked, 2-year trial of pegaptanib sodium for the treatment of diabetic macular edema. *Ophthalmology*. 2011 Jun.;118(6):1107-18.

[26] Montero, J. A., Ruiz-Moreno, J. M., De La Vega, C. Incomplete posterior hyaloid detachment after intravitreal pegaptanib injection in

diabetic macular edema. *Eur. J. Ophthalmol.* 2008 May-Jun.;18(3):469-72.

[27] Querques, G., Bux, A. V., Fusco, A. R., Iaculli, C., Delle Noci, N. Pegaptanib Sodium versus Pegaptanib Sodium Combined with Macular Laser Photocoagulation or Laser Alone for Diabetic Macular Edema. *J. Ophthalmol.* 2009;2009:672178.

[28] Morjaria, R., Chong, N. V. Pharmacokinetic evaluation of pegaptanib octasodium for the treatment of diabetic edema. *Expert Opin. Drug Metab. Toxicol.* 2014 May 24:1-8.

[29] Chun, D. W., Heier, J. S., Topping, T. M., Duker, J. S., Bankert, J. M. A pilot study of multiple intravitreal injections of ranibizumab in patients with center-involving clinically significant diabetic macular edema. *Ophthalmology*. 2006 Oct.;113(10):1706-12.

[30] Massin, P., Bandello, F., Garweg, J. G., Hansen, L. L., Harding, S. P., Larsen, M., et al. Safety and efficacy of ranibizumab in diabetic macular edema (RESOLVE Study): a 12-month, randomized, controlled, double-masked, multicenter phase II study. *Diabetes Care*. 2010 Nov.; 33 (11): 2399-405.

[31] Nguyen, Q. D., Shah, S. M., Heier, J. S., Do, D. V., Lim, J., Boyer, D., et al. Primary End Point (Six Months) Results of the Ranibizumab for Edema of the mAcula in diabetes (READ-2) study. *Ophthalmology*. 2009 Nov.;116(11):2175-81 e1.

[32] Mitchell, P., Bandello, F., Schmidt-Erfurth, U., Lang, G. E., Massin, P., Schlingemann, R. O., et al. The RESTORE study: ranibizumab monotherapy or combined with laser versus laser monotherapy for diabetic macular edema. *Ophthalmology*. 2011 Apr.;118(4):615-25.

[33] Brown, D. M., Nguyen, Q. D., Marcus, D. M., Boyer, D. S., Patel, S., Feiner, L., et al. Long-term outcomes of ranibizumab therapy for diabetic macular edema: the 36-month results from two phase III trials: RISE and RIDE. *Ophthalmology*. 2013 Oct.;120(10):2013-22.

[34] Dewan, V., Lambert, D., Edler, J., Kymes, S., Apte, R. S. Cost-effectiveness analysis of ranibizumab plus prompt or deferred laser or triamcinolone plus prompt laser for diabetic macular edema. *Ophthalmology*. 2012 Aug.;119(8):1679-84.

[35] Stein, J. D., Newman-Casey, P. A., Kim, D. D., Nwanyanwu, K. H., Johnson, M. W., Hutton, D. W. Cost-effectiveness of various interventions for newly diagnosed diabetic macular edema. *Ophthalmology*. 2013 Sep.;120(9):1835-42.

[36] Elman, M. J., Bressler, N. M., Qin, H., Beck, R. W., Ferris, F. L., 3rd, Friedman, S. M., et al. Expanded 2-year follow-up of ranibizumab plus prompt or deferred laser or triamcinolone plus prompt laser for diabetic macular edema. *Ophthalmology*. 2011 Apr.;118(4):609-14.

[37] Ollendorf, D. A., Colby, J. A., Pearson, S. D. Comparative effectiveness of anti-VEGF agents for diabetic macular edema. *Int. J. Technol. Assess. Health Care*. 2013 Oct.;29(4):392-401.

[38] Campochiaro, P. A., Wykoff, C. C., Shapiro, H., Rubio, R. G., Ehrlich, J. S. Neutralization of Vascular Endothelial Growth Factor Slows Progression of Retinal Nonperfusion in Patients with Diabetic Macular Edema. *Ophthalmology*. 2014 Apr. 23.

[39] Stewart, M. W. Critical appraisal of ranibizumab in the treatment of diabetic macular edema. *Clin. Ophthalmol*. 2013;7:1257-67.

[40] Scott, I. U., Edwards, A. R., Beck, R. W., Bressler, N. M., Chan, C. K., Elman, M. J., et al. A phase II randomized clinical trial of intravitreal bevacizumab for diabetic macular edema. *Ophthalmology*. 2007 Oct.; 114(10):1860-7.

[41] Soheilian, M., Ramezani, A., Obudi, A., Bijanzadeh, B., Salehipour, M., Yaseri, M., et al. Randomized trial of intravitreal bevacizumab alone or combined with triamcinolone versus macular photocoagulation in diabetic macular edema. *Ophthalmology*. 2009 Jun.;116(6):1142-50.

[42] Arevalo, J. F., Sanchez, J. G., Lasave, A. F., Wu, L., Maia, M., Bonafonte, S., et al. Intravitreal Bevacizumab (Avastin((R))) for Diabetic Retinopathy at 24-months: The 2008 Juan Verdaguer-Planas Lecture. *Curr. Diabetes Rev*. 2010 Sep.;6(5):313-22.

[43] Michaelides, M., Kaines, A., Hamilton, R. D., Fraser-Bell, S., Rajendram, R., Quhill, F., et al. A prospective randomized trial of intravitreal bevacizumab or laser therapy in the management of diabetic macular edema (BOLT study) 12-month data: report 2. *Ophthalmology*. 2010 Jun.;117(6):1078-86 e2.

[44] Rajendram, R., Fraser-Bell, S., Kaines, A., Michaelides, M., Hamilton, R. D., Esposti, S. D., et al. A 2-year prospective randomized controlled trial of intravitreal bevacizumab or laser therapy (BOLT) in the management of diabetic macular edema: 24-month data: report 3. *Arch. Ophthalmol*. 2012 Aug.;130(8):972-9.

[45] Sivaprasad, S., Crosby-Nwaobi, R., Heng, L. Z., Peto, T., Michaelides, M., Hykin, P. Injection frequency and response to bevacizumab monotherapy for diabetic macular oedema (BOLT Report 5). *Br. J. Ophthalmol*. 2013 Sep.;97(9):1177-80.

[46] Fortin, P., Mintzes, B., Innes, M. A systematic review of intravitreal bevacizumab for the treatment of diabetic macular edema. *CADTH Technol. Overv.* 2013;3(1):e3203.

[47] Ahmadieh, H., Ramezani, A., Shoeibi, N., Bijanzadeh, B., Tabatabaei, A., Azarmina, M., et al. Intravitreal bevacizumab with or without triamcinolone for refractory diabetic macular edema; a placebo-controlled, randomized clinical trial. *Graefes Arch. Clin. Exp. Ophthalmol.* 2008 Apr.;246(4):483-9.

[48] Solaiman, K. A., Diab, M. M., Abo-Elenin, M. Intravitreal bevacizumab and/or macular photocoagulation as a primary treatment for diffuse diabetic macular edema. *Retina.* 2010 Nov.-Dec.;30(10):1638-45.

[49] Faghihi, H., Roohipoor, R., Mohammadi, S. F., Hojat-Jalali, K., Mirshahi, A., Lashay, A., et al. Intravitreal bevacizumab versus combined bevacizumab-triamcinolone versus macular laser photocoagulation in diabetic macular edema. *Eur. J. Ophthalmol.* 2008 Nov.-Dec.;18(6):941-8.

[50] Browning, D. J., Glassman, A. R., Aiello, L. P., Beck, R. W., Brown, D. M., Fong, D. S., et al. Relationship between optical coherence tomography-measured central retinal thickness and visual acuity in diabetic macular edema. *Ophthalmology.* 2007 Mar.;114(3):525-36.

[51] Lim, J. W., Lee, H. K., Shin, M. C. Comparison of intravitreal bevacizumab alone or combined with triamcinolone versus triamcinolone in diabetic macular edema: a randomized clinical trial. *Ophthalmologica.* 2012;227(2):100-6.

[52] Marey, H. M., Ellakwa, A. F. Intravitreal bevacizumab alone or combined with triamcinolone acetonide as the primary treatment for diabetic macular edema. *Clin. Ophthalmol.* 2011;5:1011-6.

[53] Paccola, L., Costa, R. A., Folgosa, M. S., Barbosa, J. C., Scott, I. U., Jorge, R. Intravitreal triamcinolone versus bevacizumab for treatment of refractory diabetic macular oedema (IBEME study). *Br. J. Ophthalmol.* 2008 Jan.;92(1):76-80.

[54] Shahin, M. M., El-Lakkany, R. S. A prospective, randomized comparison of intravitreal triamcinolone acetonide versus intravitreal bevacizumab (avastin) in diffuse diabetic macular edema. *Middle East Afr. J. Ophthalmol.* 2010 Jul.;17(3):250-3.

[55] Ozturk, B. T., Kerimoglu, H., Bozkurt, B., Okudan, S. Comparison of intravitreal bevacizumab and ranibizumab treatment for diabetic macular edema. *J. Ocul. Pharmacol. Ther.* 2011 Aug.;27(4):373-7.

[56] Gaudreault, J., Fei, D., Rusit, J., Suboc, P., Shiu, V. Preclinical pharmacokinetics of Ranibizumab (rhuFabV2) after a single intravitreal administration. *Invest. Ophthalmol. Vis. Sci.* 2005 Feb.;46(2):726-33.

[57] Stewart, M. W., Rosenfeld, P. J. Predicted biological activity of intravitreal VEGF Trap. *Br. J. Ophthalmol.* 2008 May;92(5):667-8.

[58] Do, D. V., Nguyen, Q. D., Shah, S. M., Browning, D. J., Haller, J. A., Chu, K., et al. An exploratory study of the safety, tolerability and bioactivity of a single intravitreal injection of vascular endothelial growth factor Trap-Eye in patients with diabetic macular oedema. *Br. J. Ophthalmol.* 2009 Feb.;93(2):144-9.

[59] Do, D. V., Nguyen, Q. D., Boyer, D., Schmidt-Erfurth, U., Brown, D. M., Vitti, R., et al. One-year outcomes of the da Vinci Study of VEGF Trap-Eye in eyes with diabetic macular edema. *Ophthalmology*. 2012 Aug.;119(8):1658-65.

[60] Pareja-Rios, A., Serrano-Garcia, M. A., Marrero-Saavedra, M. D., Abraldes-Lopez, V. M., Reyes-Rodriguez, M. A., Cabrera-Lopez, F., et al. [Guidelines of clinical practice of the SERV (Spanish Retina and Vitreous Society): management of ocular complications of diabetes. Diabetic retinopathy and macular oedema]. *Arch. Soc. Esp. Oftalmol.* 2009 Sep.;84(9):429-50.

[61] *Diabetic Retinopathy Guidelines. December 2012*. The Royal College of Ophthalmologists; 2012 [9th June 2014]; Available from: http://www.rcophth.ac.uk/page.asp?section=451.

[62] Gomez-Ulla, F., Abraldes, M. J., Basauri, E., Fernandez, M., Garcia-Layana, A., Gili, P., et al. [SERV clinical practice guidelines: management of retinal vein occlusion. Sociedad Espanola de Retina y Vitreo]. *Arch. Soc. Esp. Oftalmol.* 2010 Sep.;85(9):294-309.

In: Macular Edema
Editor: Earl Davison

ISBN: 978-1-63321-584-9


*Chapter 2*

# MANAGEMENT OF MACULAR EDEMA SECONDARY TO RETINAL VEIN OCCLUSION BY INTRAVITREAL BEVACIZUMAB

***Javier A. Montero-Moreno*[1,2,*], *Jose M. Ruiz-Moreno*[3,4], *Marta Fernandez-Muñoz*[1] and *Rosa M. Sanabria-Colmenares*[5]**

[1]Pio del Rio Hortega University Hospital, Valladolid, Spain
[2]Retina Unit, Oftalvist Moncloa, Madrid, Spain
[3]Department of Ophthalmology, Castilla La Mancha University, Albacete, Spain
[4]Baviera Clinic, European Opthalmic Institute, Alicante, Spain
[5]Palencia Hospital, Palencia, Spain

## ABSTRACT

Central retinal vein occlusion (CRVO) and branch retinal vein occlusion (BRVO) are frequent causes of decreased central visual acuity (VA) related to the appearance of macular edema (ME) and ischemia. Laser treatment does not seem to improve final VA in CRVO.

* Corresponding author: Javier A. Montero Moreno. Pio Del Rio Hortega University Hospital, Ophthalmology Unit, Calle Dulzaina 2, 47012. Valladolid, Spain. Phone: +34 983 420 400. Fax: +34 983 215 365. E-mail: javiermonmor@gmail. com.

High intravitreous levels of vascular endothelial growth factor (VEGF) have been reported and therefore, intravitreous anti VEGF drugs have been used in an attempt to improve visual and anatomic outcome. Recent clinical trials have revealed the efficacy of intravitreous therapy with ranibizumab and aflibercept to reduce ME improving VA, and these drugs have been approved for such indication. Several series have reported on the efficacy of off-label intravitreous bevacizumab (IVB) to manage ME. The visual and anatomical outcome and treatment regimes of IVB in the management of ME secondary to retinal vein occlusion are discussed and compared with those results previously reported in the literature as well as the results of the main clinical trials performed with other intravitreous anti VEGF drugs.

## Introduction

Retinal vein occlusions in the form of Branch Retinal Vein Occlusion (BRVO) (Figure 1) and Central Retinal Vein Occlusion (CRVO) (Figure 2) are the most frequent vascular diseases of the retina after diabetic retinopathy (DR), affecting 1.8% and 0.5% respectively of the population aged 50 years or older [1], frequently involving the macula and resulting in low visual acuity (VA) secondary to chronic macular edema (ME), macular ischemia or damage to the retinal pigment epithelium (RPE).

CRVO typically occurs in the lamina cribrosa where the artery and the vein share a common adventitial sheath, whereas BRVO usually occurs at arterio venous crossings where the artery passes anterior to the vein.

An intermediate form of retinal vein occlusion is the hemi-central vein occlusion (H-CRVO) occurring as occlusion of only one trunk of the central retinal vein that is usually considered as a variant of CRVO.

## Pathogenesis

Histopathological studies have revealed absence of real venous compression. Instead, turbulent blood flow leads to endothelial injury and venous occlusion [2]. Even though both forms of retinal vein occlusion (RVO) may appear as perfused or non-perfused, CRVO is usually classified as ischemic or non-ischemic whereas BRVO is more frequently classified depending on the affected territory as major BRVO (affecting the major branches of the central retinal vein) or macular BRVO (in which a minor macular branch is affected causing ME with decreased VA).

The pathogenesis of CRVO and BRVO is still unclear though it is known to be related to a relative reduction of retinal vein lumen, leading to the Virchow triad formed by reduced blood flow, increased blood viscosity and damage to the endothelial cells.

In most cases hemorrhage, edema and ischemia are caused by the reduced venous flow associated with increased intracapillary hydrostatic pressure and microvascular closure with leukocytes in the territory of the affected vessel.

Retinal vein occlusions affect more frequently patients older than 65, especially those with arterial hypertension, smoking, diabetes mellitus, dyslipidemia and higher body mass index, as well as neoplasia and vasculitis. The appearance of RVO among younger patients is more frequently associated with thrombophilia.

According to a meta-analysis study performed by O'Mahoney, the most frequently found factors are arterial hypertension (63% vs. 36% in controls) followed by hyperlipidemia [3].

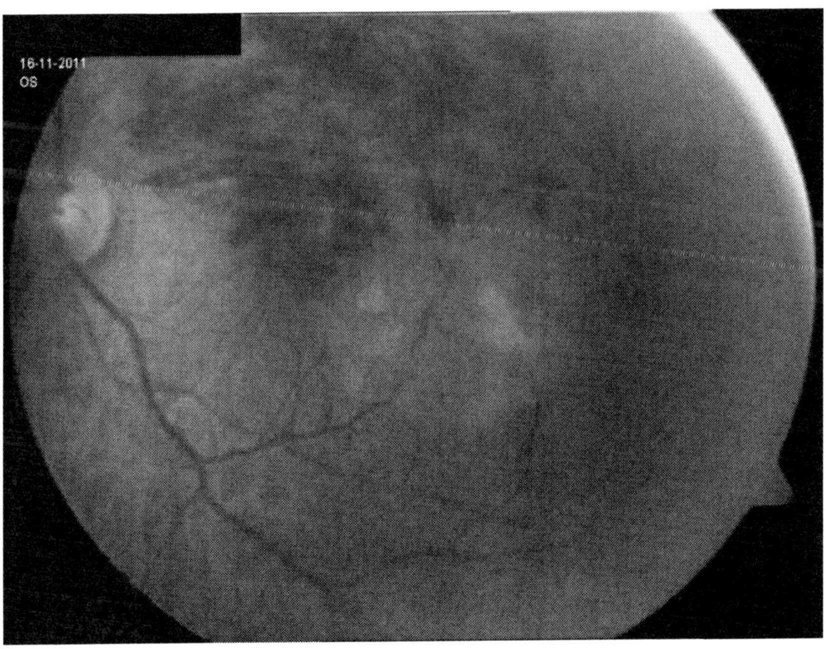


Figure 1. Temporal superior branch retinal vein occlusion (BRVO) with macular edema (ME), retinal hemorrhages and cotton-wool spots corresponding to ischemic areas.

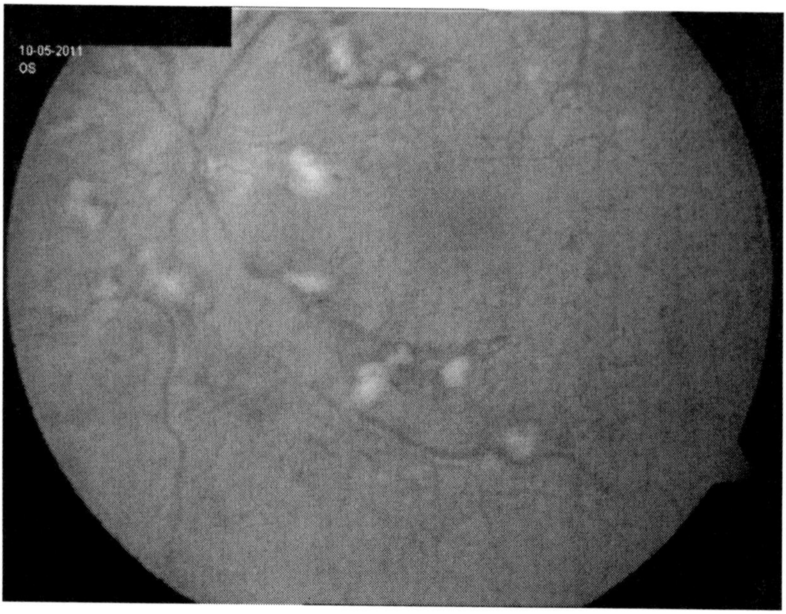


Figure 2. Central retinal vein occlusion with flame-shaped retinal hemorrhages affecting four quadrants and retinal ischemia as shown by the presence of multiple cotton wool spots.

Hyperopia, atherosclerosis and hypertension seem to be more frequent in BRVO, whereas glaucoma is more frequent in CRVO.

RVO may cause decreased VA secondary to ME and ischemia, as well as retinal and vitreous hemorrhage, retinal detachment and neovascular glaucoma (NVG) with anterior segment neovascularization. The prognosis of BRVO is usually good with most of the eyes achieving a final VA ≥65 Early Treatment Diabetic Retinopathy Study (ETDRS) letters spontaneously. According to a study performed by Rehak et al. on eyes with BRVO, visual prognosis is good in eyes with initial VA ≥65 letters. In their series most of the eyes with initial VA <35 letters ended with VA ≤35 letters [4]. Most of the eyes with non-ischemic CRVO achieved final VA ≥70 letters without any treatment and lower initial VA and larger ischemic areas correlated with poorer final VA.

## TREATMENT

Several different therapeutic options have been proposed for the management of ME secondary to RVO.

Among the therapies that have been explored for the treatment of RVO, and have failed to achieve the desired results or were associated with severe side effects complications, are: laser-induced chorioretinal anastomosis, intravitreal recombinant tissue plasminogen activator (rTPA), isovolemic hemodilution, oral pentoxifylline, hyperbaric oxygen therapy and surgery (radial optic neurotomy (RON), sheathotomy, vitrectomy with or without internal limiting membrane peeling and direct injection of rTPA into the lumen of the occluded retinal vein) [5-9].

The Branch Retinal Vein Occlusion Study (BRVO Study) recommended grid argon laser photocoagulation in eyes with ME and VA <70 letters [10], whereas in CRVO laser treatment did not show any visual benefit [11]. Intravitreous injections of steroids (triamcinolone acetonide (TA) [12, 13], dexamethasone [14] and flucinolone [15]) have shown therapeutic benefits reducing ME and improving VA, even though they are frequently associated with moderate to severe side effects such as increased intraocular pressure (IOP) and cataracts.

During the past few years varied intravitreous anti vascular endothelial growth factor (anti-VEGF) drugs have become available and been used in the management of ME secondary to retinal vascular conditions such as diabetic retinopathy, BRVO and CRVO with promising results.

## Role of Vascular Endothelial Growth Factor

The ischemic retina releases different cytokines. Green et al. proved the presence of ischemic changes in the internal retina in eyes enucleated for CRVO [16]. Funk et al. reported on cytokine concentrations in eyes with CRVO and BRVO, finding that aqueous samples of eyes with CRVO showed significantly increased levels of VEGF, interleukins (IL) IL-6, IL-8, IP-10, monocyte chemotactic protein (MCP)-1 and platelet derived growth factor (PDGF)-AA compared with the control samples [17].

Koss et al. evaluated the concentrations of cytokines (IL-6, MCP-1 and VEGFA) in undiluted vitreous of patients with ME secondary to BRVO, CRVO and H-CRVO. The mean cytokine values were highest in the CRVO group followed by the H-CRVO group and the BRVO groups, and all values were significantly higher than in the control samples [18].

Noma et al. found increased vitreous and aqueous concentrations of VEGF and IL-6 that were significantly correlated with the non-perfused area of BRVO and with the severity of ME [19].

Furthermore, intravitreous injections of VEGF induce retinal changes similar to those found in eyes with CRVO and proliferative diabetic retinopathy (PDR) such as retinal ischemia, and hemorrhages and retinal edema [20]. The intravitreous concentration of VEGF varies among the different studies and retinal conditions, but it is generally accepted that is highest in CRVO, followed by PDR, BRVO and exudative age related macular degeneration (AMD), explaining why ME is harder to manage in eyes with CRVO [21].

VEGF is formed by several isomers that can be subdivided into 5 different subgroups (VEGFA, VEGFB, VEGFC, VEGFD, and placental growth factor, PlGF); among them VEGFA is the key regulator of physiologic and pathologic angiogenesis. Among the different VEGFA isoforms ($VEGFA_{121}$, $VEGFA_{146}$, $VEGFA_{165}$, $VEGFA_{183}$, $VEGFA_{189}$ and $VEGFA_{206}$), $VEGFA_{165}$ is the most common and the most important for angiogenesis. VEGF activates three membrane-spanning tyrosin kinases (VEGFR-1, VEGFR-2 and VEGFR-3) (membrane receptors).

VEGFR-1 induces matrix metalloproteinases, releases tissue specific growth factors, and recruits endothelial progenitors and VEGFR-2 mediates in the permeability enhancing and angiogenic effect of VEGFR-1. VEGF is produced by the RPE, pericytes, astrocytes, neurons, endothelial cells, ganglion cells, Müller cells and smooth muscle cells; and the cellular targets of VEGF (that is, cells expressing VEGFR-2) are the endothelial cells of the choroid and the retina, ganglion cells, Müller cells, RPE and photoreceptors.

The most common cause of increased VEGF synthesis is tissue hypoxia [22], even though intraocular inflammation can up-regulate the synthesis of VEGF messenger RNA through certain mediator molecules such as epidermal growth factor, transforming growth factor (TGF)-$\alpha$ and -$\beta$, insulin-like growth factor 1, fibroblast growth factor (FGF), IL-1$\alpha$, IL-6, protein-kinase C-$\beta$ and PDGF [23].

Among the effects of VEGF as a growth and survival factor, VEGF stimulates the mitosis and swelling of arterial and venous endothelial cells, thus initiating angiogenesis [24].

Vasodilation induced by dose-dependent nitric oxid release and fenestration across cell bodies accompanied by dissolution of intercellular tight junctions induced by metalloproteinases facilitates fluid outflow from the retinal capillaries into the retina [25-28].

Therefore, blockade of the VEGF effects seems a reasonable approach for the management of ME related to RVO.

## ANTIANGIOGENIC TREATMENT

Presently several antiangiogenic molecules are available for intravitreous injection in the management of vascular retinal conditions.

Pegaptanib sodium (Macugen®, Pfizer) is a synthetic 40kD RNA aptamer that binds specifically to the $VEGF_{165}$ isoform and was approved as intravitreous injection for the management of exudative AMD. Pegaptanib was tried to reduce ME in patients with CRVO and BRVO though it was not approved for this indication. Wroblewski et al. evaluated the efficacy of two different dosages of pegaptanib to reduce ME in patients with CRVO in a group of 33 patients vs. a similar control group treated by sham injections, observing a significant reduction of central macular thickness (CMT)CMT as well as better VA outcome in treated eyes at six months [29]. Similar outcomes were reported after a prospective non-controlled study at 1 year in eyes with BRVO [30].

Ranibizumab (Lucentis®, Genetech, Hoffmann-La RocheNovartis) is an anti-VEGF agent formed by a modified Fab fraction of a humanized monoclonal antibody that was initially tried for exudative AMD and was later successfully ustried to treat ME in patients with diabetic retinopathy and RVO. Ranibizumab shows a high affinity for VEGFA. The largest study performed to evaluate its efficacy in BRVO was the BRAVO trial, in which 397 patients were randomized to receive grid laser, monthly intravitreous 0.3 or 0.5mg ranibizumab (IVR) or both treatments [31-33]. At six months, most of the patients treated by IVR showed a VA gain of 15 letters or more vs. 29% of the patients in the control group, and the average VA gain in the first group was 16.6 to 18.3 letters vs. 7.3 letters in the group treated by the standard of care (grid laser photocoagulation or observation). The CRUISEruise study evaluated 392 patients with ME secondary to CRVO, randomized to 0.3 or 0.5mg of IVR or sham injections. Treated eyes showed an average VA gain of 12.7 to 14.9 letters at month 6 vs. 0. 8 in the sham group, with almost 50% of the treated eyes achieving 15 or more letters gained at month 6 vs. 17% in the sham group [34]. The HORIZON study evaluated the results of 608 patients from the BRAVO and the CRUISE studies at 1 year in order to assess the appearance of safety events. Even though no new safety events appeared after 1 year, reduced follow-up and fewer injections during the second year of treatment resulted in a decline of VA in CRVO patients with stabilization of VA in BRVO eyes [33].

Aflibercept or VEGF Trap-Eye (Eylea®, Bayer) is a synthetic fusion protein consisting of domain 2 of VEGFR1 and domain 3 of VEGFR2 fused with an Fc-IgG backbone that acts as a decoy receptor, binding and inhibiting VEGFA as well as VEGFB and PlGF with a higher affinity than ranibizumab. A multicenter study randomized 189 patients with ME secondary to CRVO to 2mg intravitreous aflibercept or sham. At week 24, 56% of the treated patients gained 15 or more letters vs. 30% of the sham group and this improvement was maintained at 1 year [35].

The results of the Copernicus and the Galileo studies on the use of intravitreal aflibercept to treat ME related to CRVO have been recently released [36, 37]. Both trials were designed to evaluate the efficacy and safety of intravitreal aflibercept injections for the treatment of ME secondary to CRVO on 189 and 167 patients, respectively. One of the characteristics of these trials that made them significantly different from previous trials is that patients with retinal ischemia were not excluded. Patients were randomized to be treated by intravitreal injections of 2mg aflibercept every 4 weeks or sham during 6 months. Afterwards, both groups of patients in the Copernicus trial were treated on a *pro re nata* (PRN) regime with aflibercept until week 52, as well as those in the Galileo active treatment group, whereas those in the sham group in the Galileo study were treated by sham injections on a PRN regime until week 52. Photocoagulation was allowed as rescue therapy in both studies. The demographics of both studies did not differ significantly from those of the CRUISE trial apart from the fact that ischemic patients were included.

VA improved in the active treatment arms after the first injection and reached a plateau after the third injection and until week 24 (+17.3/+18.0 letters, for Copernicus and Galileo, respectively), or showed a mild spontaneous improvement (+3.3 letters for Galileo) or decrease (-4.0 letters for Copernicus) in the sham treated group by week 24.

Interestingly, the prevalence of ischemia in the sham group of the Copernicus trial was higher (16.4%) than in Galileo (10.3%), what might account for the VA loss in the untreated group of Galileo.

Active treatment during the second semester in the Copernicus trial permitted a mild VA improvement in the previously non-treated group (+3.8 from baseline, +7.8 letters from VA at week 24) with stabilization of VA in the same group of the Galileo trial that remained on sham treatment (+3.8 from baseline, + 0.3 letters from VA at week 24).

During the second year active treatment was performed PRN with very small differences in both trials (Copernicus, +13.0 and +1.5 letters from baseline for the active treatment and sham group, respectively; Galileo +13.7 and +6.2 from baseline for the active treatment and sham group, respectively). WInterestingly, when eyes with and without ischemia were compared, it was observed that VA gain did not differ significantly between ischemic and perfused eyes in the active treatment arms.

However, VA loss was deeper among ischemic eyes than among perfused eyes in the sham treatment arm, and VA improvement after treatment was higher among ischemic eyes. Similarly, reduction in central macular thickness (CMT) by week 24 was more pronounced in aflibercept treated eyes (-457.2 and -448.6μm) than in the sham treated eyes (-144.8 and -166.0). 60% of the treated eyes gained ≥15 ETDRS letters by week 24. The safety profile was good in both trials with 1 or less local severe adverse events (except for ME), and no differences in cardiovascular events except for arterial hypertension, that was more frequent among treated eyes (14.9% vs. 9.5%).

Bevacizumab (Avastin®, Hoffmann-La Roche) is a full-length humanized monoclonal antibody that binds all forms of VEGFA, and was primarily indicated and approved to be used systemically to treat metastasized cancers, even though due to its lower price when used intravitreously compared to other intravitreous drugs, and its availability it has been used extensively off-label to treat ME associated with BRVO and CRVO, as well as diabetic ME and exudative AMD. Even though they share a common origin, bevacizumab and ranibizumab are different molecules, with different pharmacokinetics and power to block VEGF. Since bevacizumab is not intended for intraocular issue, local and systemic safety has been a concern until recent prospective comparative studies (CATT [38, 39], IVAN [40]. MANTA [41]) have shown a similar safety profile for bevacizumab and ranibizumab. The half-life of intravitreal bevacizumab (IVB) is longer than that of IVR. [42]. Therefore, the recommended dosing interval for IVR for BRVO and CRVO (four weeks, according to the BRAVO and CRUISE studies) [33] may not be the same as for IVB, permitting up to six weeks intervals between injections.

## Intravitreous Bevacizumab in BRVO

Several studies have been performed in order to evaluate the efficacy and safety of IVB in ME secondary to BRVO showing improvement in VA and CMT. Most of the studies used 1.25 and 2.5mg IVB, even though it seems that there are no significant differences between both dosages at 2 years, as was found by the Pan-American Collaborative Retina Study [43, 44].

However, since anti VEGF treatment addresses only one of the secondary pathogenic mechanisms that lead to the appearance of ME and neovascularization and does not address the causes of RVO, rebounds are the rule and regular repeated injections are required.

In order to avoid this inconvenience, IVB has been combined with other therapies such as grid laser photocoagulation [45].

IVB has been compared with grid laser photocoagulation, finding that even though both treatments improved VA and CMT, the benefits were larger in the IVB group [46].

Hikichi et al. evaluated the effects of IVB on 89 treatment-naïve eyes with ME secondary to BRVO that were followed during 2 years after IVB. In this series the mean number of injections was 2.6±0.9 during the first year and 1.3±1.0 during the second year. 13% of the eyes did not require further treatment after the first injection, and 26% of the eyes required rescue laser therapy [47]. It is likely that those eyes that required only one injection might have showed some spontaneous improvement of ME without any treatment; however, no definite data can predict the eyes in which ME will resolve during the natural disease course and it has been shown that a shorter duration of ME is associated with greater improvement after treatment [12].

The effect of IVB has also been compared with intravitreal triamcinolone (IVT). Gokce et al. compared both treatment modalities in eyes with ME secondary to BRVO with and without macular ischemia. A larger improvement in CMT and VA was observed among the eyes treated by IVT during the early period even though the differences were no longer significant at one year. This difference was more evident in non-ischemic eyes [48]. The number of injections required was also significantly higher in eyes treated by IVB, and the amount of ocular complications was higher for the eyes treated by IVT, mainly cataracts and increased IOP.

The comparative efficacy of IVB and IVR has been evaluated by several groups., such as the study performed by Yuan et al. who retrospectively compared 26 eyes treated with IVR, 33 eyes with IVB, and 22 eyes with IVB then switched to IVR (crossover) [49].

This series showed a trend favoring IVR vs. IVB in terms of VA gain at 6 weeks and 2 months even though without statistical significance.

No differences were observed in terms of reduction of CMT. Switching from IVB to IVR improved anatomic outcome in some eyes with cystoid ME, though the functional change was not significant.

Kumagai compared the efficacy of vitrectomy with IVB and intravitreous rTPA. The three treatments appeared to provide similar visual outcomes at 12 months without significant differences, even though repeated injections of both drugs wereas required [50]. Combined IVB and grid laser photocoagulation maintain VA improvement with limited effects on further recurrences of ME, resulting in a reduced number of injections compared with IVB monotherapy.

Ehrlich et al. combined IVB with intravitreous TA, finding that combined treatment improved structural outcome, with no additional advantages over IVB monotherapy [51].

Yilmaz et al. performed a systematic review to assess the effectiveness of IVB in the treatment of ME associated with BRVO [52].

Four trials were revised comparing IVB with a control group, showing VA and CMT improvement at 12 weeks.

Singer et al. performed a retrospective study on patients with CRVO and BRVO treated by IVR and IVB followed by an intravitreous dexamethasone implant two weeks later. Both groups of treatment achieved a significant CMT decrease with VA improvement by week 2 and week 6, even though both VA and CMT improvement was significantly greater in eyes treated by IVR vs. IVB [21]. The authors attributed these differences to the higher affinity of ranibizumab for VEGF, as well as the higher intraocular concentration of VEGF in CRVO and BRVO compared with exudative AMD, and the very short-term data.

We have performed a retrospective study on 32 eyes with BRVO, that were treated with monthly IVB at least one month after detection of decreased vision related to BRVO on a PRN regime. Fifteen of them were males and 17 females. The mean age was 70±9 years. Mean baseline VA was 44.5±20.0 ETDRS letters, and the mean baseline CMT was 592±242μm. One year after the initial IVB was performed, VA was 58.0±21.9 ($p=0.009$, Student t test). The average number of injections performed was 4.3±2.4. During the 2$^{nd}$ and 3$^{rd}$ years an average 1.8±2.2 and 2.1±2.4 IVB were performed. The number of injections performed ranged from 1 to 11 during the 1$^{st}$ year, from 0 to 8 during the 2$^{nd}$ year and 0 to 7 during the 3$^{rd}$ year. CMT averaged 313±173μm at 1 year and 300±150μm at 2 years ($p=0.0004$ and 0.0007 respectively; Student t test).

VA gain was maintained at 2 and 3 years (64.3±17.5, $p=0.004$). None of the cases presented severe local or systemic adverse events. No eyes required laser treatment or presented *rubeosis iridis* during follow-up. There were two eyes that still required almost monthly intravitreal injections during the 4$^{th}$ year; these eyes presented neovascular shunts that connected the obstructed vein branch with healthy vessels, despite the continuous anti-VEGF treatment (Figures 3 and 4).

The optimal dosing schedule for IVB in eyes with ME secondary to BRVO has not been established. Monthly initial injections seem to be effective as shown for ranibizumab in the BRAVO trial, though they are frequently inconvenient for patients, ophthalmologists and for the Health Services.

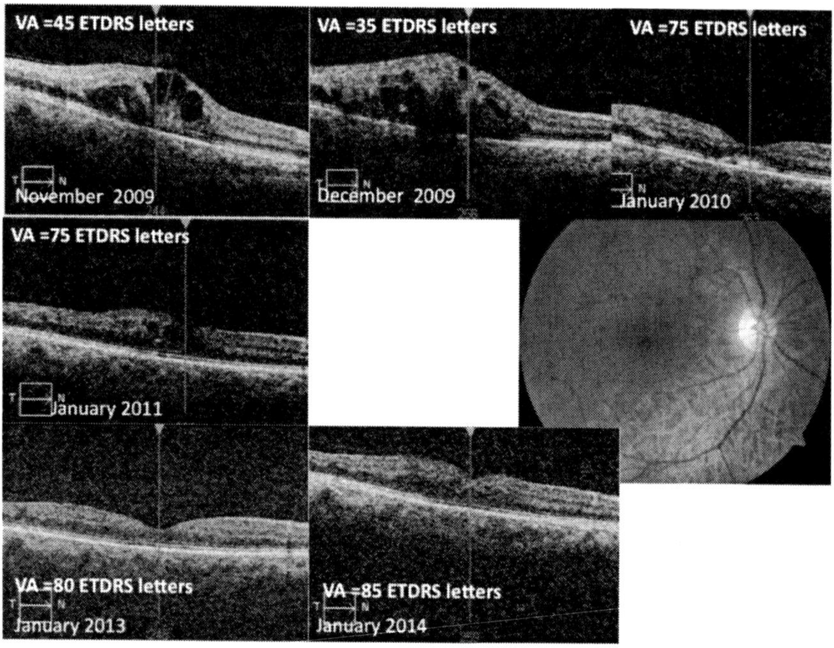


Figure 3. Temporal superior BRVO with macular edema as shown by optical coherence tomography (OCT). After BRVO diagnosis (Top left) the patient remained under observation during one month, and ME worsening was observed (top center). Intravitreal bevacizumab (IVB) was started on a monthly regime and central macular thickness decreased as shown in the following OCT images (notice the date in the bottom of each image). Center bottom: The final OCT image (January 2014) corresponds to the retinal photograph shown at center, right. Visual acuity is shown in ETDRS letters.

Therefore it has been considered that a three-monthly regime might be a practical alternative. Ahn et al. have demonstrated that there are no statistical difference in VA or CMT results between a PRN regime and 3 monthly initial doses followed by PRN injections for 6 months and at 1 year [53], suggesting that PRN IVB is more tolerable for patients with ME secondary to BRVO.

## INTRAVITREOUS BEVACIZUMAB IN CRVO

In 2005 Rosenfeld et al. evaluated the effects of 1mg IVB on VA and optical coherence tomography (OCT) in one patient with ME resulting from CRVO. The patient had been previously treated by IVT that had resulted in VA improvement associated with cataracts and increased IOP. One week after the IVB, VA improved from 35 to 65 ETDRS letters and OCT revealed resolution of ME.

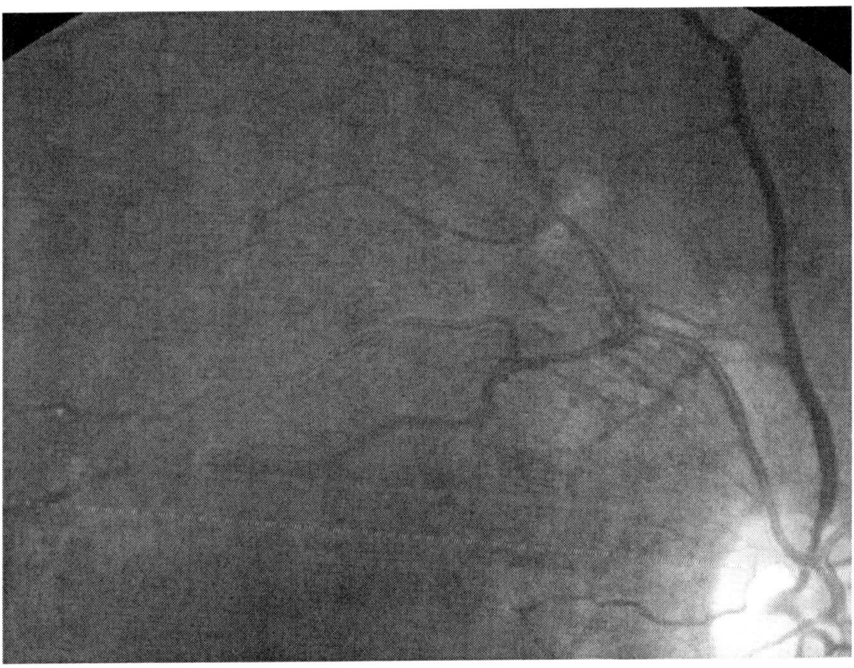

Figure 4. Enlarged detail of the retinal photograph in Figure 3, shows the presence of collateral vessels connecting the obstructed temporal superior vein with healthy vessels after 4 years of monthly IVB.

One week after the IVB, VA improved from 35 to 65 ETDRS letters and OCT revealed resolution of ME.

Ferrara et al. [54] retrospectively evaluated visual and retinal changes in 6 eyes from 5 patients with CRVO treated by IVB (ranging from 4 to 10 injections) within the first three months of the occlusion, and followed during 12 months [54]. Baseline VA was 18 ETDRS letters and 64 letters at the last follow-up visit, with a significant decrease in optic nerve head swelling and venous diameter and tortuosity. The largest proportion of improvement occurred within one month of the first injection.

Shortly afterwards, in 2007 the German Retina Society assessed what treatment methods were preferred for CRVO among its members, finding that 64% of them recommended isovolemic hemodilution, 32% pentoxifylline infusions and 43% advised RON. However, most of the 124 respondents (72%) applied intravitreal anti-VEGF treatment, and the majority of them (94%) used IVB.

Since then, more than 70 papers have been published on the use of IVB. In 2007 Prigingler reported on a large series of 46 patients with CRVO treated by 1.25mg IVB in a prospective, interventional case series [55]. Mean VA improved from 30 ETDRS letters at baseline to 55 at the 6-month follow-up associated with decreased CMT from 535±148μm to 323±116μm at the 6-month follow-up. Ischemic forms were associated with lower baseline and final VA, though VA gain was similar in both groups.

Moschos et al. [56] evaluated the effectiveness and toxicity of IVB in the management of ME related to CRVO on 10 patients by multifocal electroretinography (MFERG) and OCT after 1 and 3 months follow-up. They observed increased CMT before treatment that decreased to a significant level at 1 and 3 months after treatment.

The electrical responses in the fovea and parafovea depicted a significant improvement at 1 and 3 months after the injection.

Epstein et al. [57] reported on a prospective, randomized, double-masked trial to evaluate the efficacy of IVB to treat ME secondary to CRVO on 60 patients. Patients were randomized to receive either IVB or sham injections every 6 weeks for 6 months. Eighteen of 30 patients in the study group gained ≥15 ETDRS letters compared with 6 of 30 patients in the control group ($p=0.003$). In the treated group average VA improved by 14.1 letters compared with a decrease of 2.0 letters in the control group ($p< 0.003$), and the mean CMT decrease was significantly greater in the study group (426μm) compared with the control group (102μm). *Rubeosis iridis* was observed in 5 of 30 patients in the sham group vs. no cases in the study group ($p=0.052$). The authors reported no local or systemic severe adverse events in either group, concluding that IVB given every 6 weeks was a safe treatment, improving VA and reducing ME.

Pikkel et al. [58] revised a series of 68 patients treated for ischemic CRVO with IVB in order to assess injection protocols on final VA. Thirty-nine patients had been treated by a preset protocol of one monthly injection during three consecutive months, and 29 by one single intravitreal injection (six of them received one further injection and two of them received two further injections). Patients treated with one single injection as initial protocol were compared to patients treated with three injections, and the effect of the timing of the first injection on the final visual outcome was evaluated, showing that IVB applied up to 3 months following CRVO improved VA.

Early first injection and multiple injections had a positive effect on final VA, though treatment timing had a greater effect than the number of injections administered.

Patients treated by only one early IVB within 1 month of diagnosis showed a better final VA than those who were treated by three IVB more than 2 months after the diagnosis, and the difference was almost statistically significant ($p = 0.063$). Patients treated by one single injection followed by additional injections applied later showed less improvement than those treated by a preset protocol of three injections. Similarly, intravitreal injections performed more than three months after the CRVO episode were not effective. The authors concluded that VA improved after IVB in ME related to CRVO, and this improvement was greater among those in whom the first injection was given early and in those cases in which three injections were administered in a scheduled regime.

In order to evaluate the efficacy and safety of the anti-VEGF therapies in the management of ME related to CRVO, Huang et al. [59] performed a meta-analysis study based on five clinical trials consisting of 323 cases and 281 controls, eliminating between-study heterogeneity. The results showed that an overall comparison of anti-VEGF therapies with placebo control yielded a 374% and 136% increased tendency for a gain ≥15 ETDRS letters with these treatments ($p=0.00001$ and $p=0.0001$) at 6 and 12 month, respectively. Similarly, the risk of losing ≥15 ETDRS letters was decreased by 90% and 77% at 6 and 12 months. Changes of CMT were no longer significant at 12 months after 6 month PRN treatment. Interestingly, the incidence of adverse events showed no statistical difference between anti-VEGF and placebo groups. Considering the different drugs used, aflibercept got the best tendency to gain ≥15 letters, followed by bevacizumab and the best tendency to reduced CMT was observed for with aflibercept and ranibizumab.

The chances of improving VA were better in patients aged <50 years, and in eyes with ischemic CRVO.

We have performed a retrospective study on 19 eyes from 19 patients with CRVO and H-CRVO, including ischemic and non-ischemic vein occlusions. Thirteen patients were males. The eyes were treated by PRN IVB at least one month after decreased VA was diagnosed. The mean age was 67±13 years.

Mean baseline VA was 30.0±24.1 ETDRS letters with an average CMT of 732±204μm. By the end of the first year and after an average 6.3±3.1 IVB, VA was 51.4±25.0 letters (p= 0.01, Student t for paired data) and CMT was 442±303μm (p= 0.01). (Figure 5) During the 2nd and 3rd year, an average of 5.4±3.6 and 5.2±4.4 injections were performed respectively, for an average VA of 45.9.5±26.9 and 56.2±21.8 ETDRS letters respectively (p= 0.1 and p= 0.02, respectively) and an average CMT of 451±359 and 554±275μm respectively (p= 0.04 and p= 0.02, respectively).

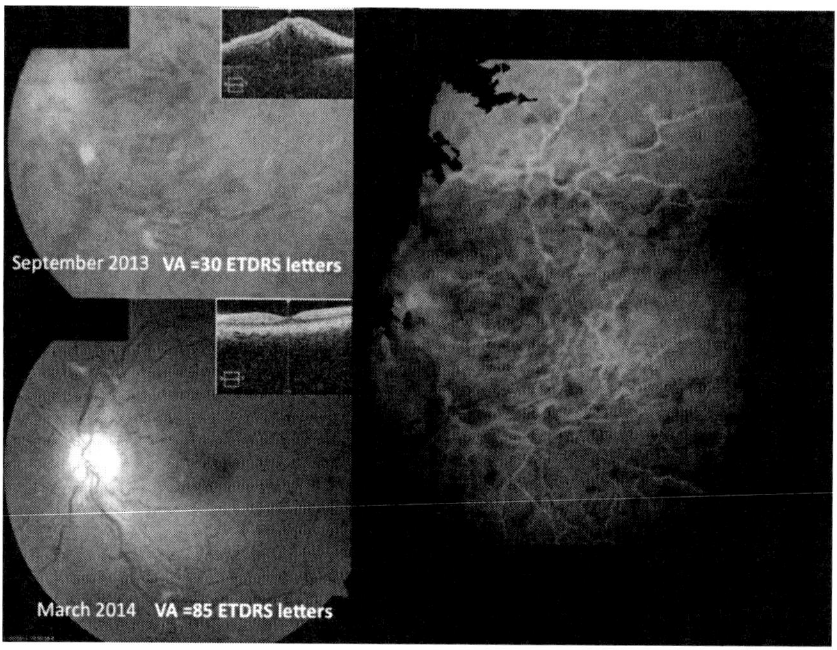


Figure 5. Top left: Fundus photograph and OCT in a case of central retinal vein occlusion (CRVO) and OCT (inset) with ME and VA=30 ETDRS letters. Top right: Fluorescein angiography (FA) shows multiple retinal hemorrhages with ischemia and ME. Bottom left: After 4 months of treatment with IVB, and 2 months treatment-free, ME is completely resolved with VA=85 letters.

One eye presented *rubeosis iridis* at baseline that disappeared with treatment. No eyes required laser treatment or presented *rubeosis iridis* during follow-up.

None of the patients presented local or systemic severe adverse events, including NVG.

All the eyes presented optic disk shunts after the second year similar to those found after RON, despite the frequent use of intravitreal antiangiogenic drugs (ranging 0 to 13 injections per year) (Figures 6 and 7).

## ANTI-VEGF IN ISCHEMIC RETINA

A growing corpus of data has become available during the past decade on the efficacy and safety of intravitreal anti-VEGF therapy in eyes with ME secondary to retinal vascular disease, as suggested by good visual outcomes. However, patients with ischemic retina have been frequently excluded from the main clinical trials, since visual prognosis might be substantially worse in these eyes. It has been reported that IVR may induce arterial vasoconstriction in eyes with exudative AMD, which might worsen retinal ischemia in RVO [60].

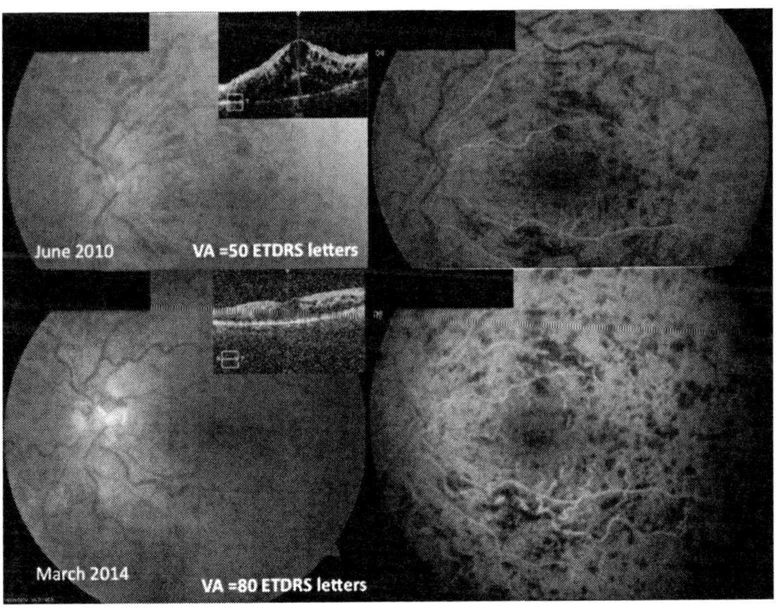


Figure 6. Top left: Fundus photograph and OCT in a case of CRVO. OCT shows ME with VA=50 ETDRS letters. Top right and bottom right: FA shows multiple retinal hemorrhages with ME. Bottom left: After almost four years of monthly IVB, ME is resolved and VA is 80 ETDRS letters. Notice the presence of multiple vascular shunts in the optic disk.

However, patients with ischemic retina have been frequently excluded from the main clinical trials, since visual prognosis might be substantially worse in these eyes.

It has been reported that IVR may induce arterial vasoconstriction in eyes with exudative AMD, which might worsen retinal ischemia in RVO [60].

Spaide et al. evaluated retinal ischemia by means of wide field FA in eyes treated by IVR for CRVO, detecting large confluent non-perfused areas in the peripheral retina in all the cases [61].

These new techniques have provided new research tools that are changing our idea of non-perfused RVO, since peripheral areas of non-perfused retina did not differ significantly among eyes that would have been classified as non-perfused according to the CRVO Study imaging criteria and those that would have been considered as perfused.

These authors did not find any correlation between the number of injections performed and increased non-perfused areas.

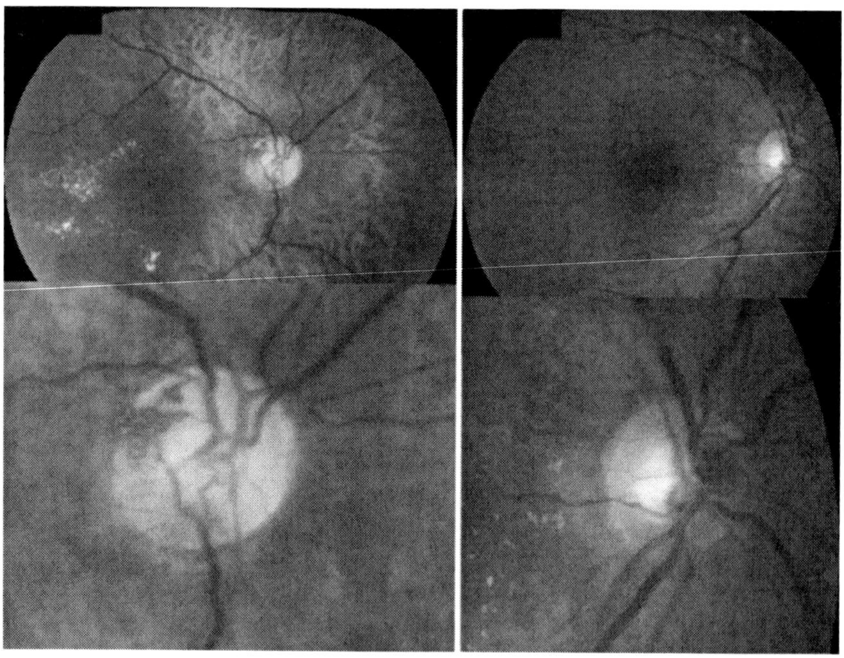

Figure 7. Two cases of CRVO after treatment with IVB showing optic disk shunts.

The BRAVO and the CRUISE studies were not performed on patients with ischemic areas larger than 10 disk diameters, and 12 month worsening of macular ischemia was not reported as an adverse event, even though the authors did not exclude it either.

Manousaridis and Talks have performed a literature search on the possible effect of anti-VEGF therapy on the ischemic retina [62]. The degree of ischemia was evaluated in most of the studies on the basis of fluorescein angiography, even though most of the studies lacked an adequate uniform gradation of macular ischemia. The authors concluded that the question whether macular ischemia may be aggravated by sustained anti-VEGF treatment remains open; the efficacy and safety of these therapies has been proved, though worsening of macular ischemia cannot be excluded, and suggest that eyes with severe capillary loss according to ETDRS criteria or a foveal avascular zone >1000 μm should be considered as having severe ischemia, making it necessary to evaluate periodically the macular condition by FA, and not only by OCT.

Collateral vessels are considered to be a desirable event in patients with RVO compensating for the poor flow in the obstructed vessels.

Collaterals at the optic disk have been described in 77% of the cases with CRVO [63]. It has been hypothesized that restoration of venous flow in RVO occurs by recanalization of the obstructed vessel or by the development of collateral vessels, and VEGF has the capacity of promoting the formation of collateral vessels. Bevacizumab and ranibizumab are non-selective VEGF blockers that may down-regulate the normal physiological functions of VEGF, and it has been suggested that sustained VEGF inhibition might increase neuroretinal apoptosis and/ or capillary dropout, eventually worsening visual function by impairing re-perfusion of occluded capillaries and development of collaterals, and inducing vasoconstriction of the normal capillaries, reducing retinal blood flow supply [62]. Ferrara et al. did not observe collateral vessels at the optic nerve head in the mentioned series on patients with CRVO treated by IVB [54]. However, in our series on BRVO and CRVO with longer follow-up treated by monthly IVB, those eyes with BRVO and CRVO that required maintained treatment developed collateral vessels. Ferrara found VA improvement lacking retinal re-perfusion difficult to explain. We consider that even though IVB helps preventing macular damage secondary to ME in eyes with RVO, the limited half life of IVB and the high production of VEGF in the ischemic retina may give way to a slow but progressive appearance of vessels in the retinal surface though they will not give way to a fibrovascular proliferation or distant neovascularization. Due to the appearance of irreversible neural damage in eyes with sustained ME, that is secondary not only to macular ischemia but also to the elongation and rupture of photoreceptors, we consider that intravitreal anti VEGF therapy should be started promptly, in cases where the natural course of the disease is towards progressive ME. This finding is reinforced by the appearance of intraretinal neovascularization and shunts in eyes with CRVO and BRVO that is not prevented by the intravitreal administration of anti-VEGF drugs. This treatment should be performed and maintained on a regular schedule every 4 to 6 weeks in order to maintain a dry macula, and its frequency can be slightly changed according to the appearance of macular changes and VA.

# Treatment Protocols

## Spanish Vitreo Retina Society

The Spanish Vitreo Retina Society recommends the following algorithm for the management of ME secondary to RVO (Table 1) [64].

**Table 1. Spanish Vitreo Retina Society algorithm for the management of ME secondary to retinal vein occlusion [64]**

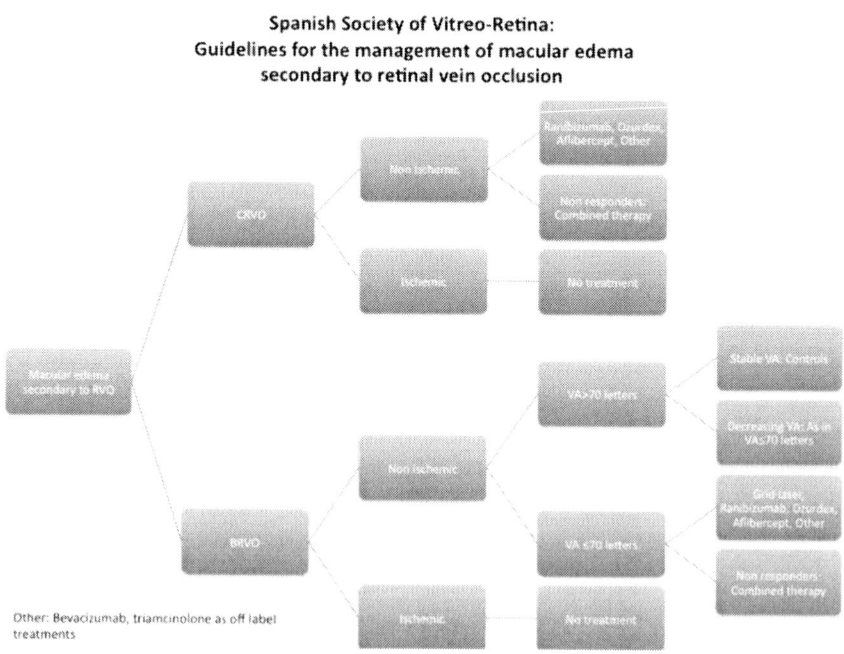

## Conclusion

In comparative studies, all anti-VEGF treatments have achieved a higher VA improvement vs. steroids at month 12 in eyes with ME secondary to CRVO. Continuous IVB every 6 weeks achieved +16 ETDRS letters gain [65] vs. +13.4 letters gain after IVR every 4 weeks during the first three months followed by PRN regime [66]. Best VA gain has been reported for IVR in the BRAVO trial at month 12 after 0.5mg ranibizumab, performed monthly for 6 months followed by monthly PRN resulting in +18.3 letters after an average 8.4 injections [67]. IVB studies achieved similar results (+15 to +17 letters) with a much lower number of participants [46, 68]. The rate of ocular adverse events was very low in all the evaluated studies and the frequency of endophthalmitis was under 1% regardless of the drug used. Even though increased IOP has been occasionally reported in eyes treated by intravitreal anti-VEGF drugs, none of the eyes in the reported series required treatment for high IOP.

Systemic risks were similarly low for all the treatments, and the rates of death were very low (0-3%) with no statistically significant differences for the different drugs. No significant differences were found for cerebrovascular events or non-ocular hemorrhages or infections.

Hahn et al. advocate intravitreal anti VEGF agents for the management of ME secondary to RVO as a first line therapy, reserving intravitreal steroids for pseudophakic unresponsive patients due to the high risk of ocular side effects associated with steroids. Grid laser can be performed for consolidation of the results [69].

The same paradigm applies for ME in CRVO eyes; in these cases intravitreal anti VEGF therapy and steroids can be used.

However, the risk of overlooking NVG in steroid treated patients with high IOP should be born in mind, especially since intravitreal steroids do not block anterior chamber neovascularization and increased IOP secondary to NVG can be mistaken with steroid-induced high IOP.

Even though IVR has been established as the new gold-standard for BRVO against grid laser photocoagulation, small trials implicate similar outcomes for IVB. Head to head trials similar to those previously performed for exudative AMD are required to evaluate the superiority or similar efficacy of IVB.

## REFERENCES


[1] Klein, R., Moss, S. E., Meuer, S. M., Klein, B. E. The 15-year cumulative incidence of retinal vein occlusion: the Beaver Dam Eye Study. *Arch. Ophthalmol.* 2008 Apr.;126(4):513-8.

[2] Jefferies, P., Clemett, R., Day, T. An anatomical study of retinal arteriovenous crossings and their role in the pathogenesis of retinal branch vein occlusions. *Aust. N. Z. J. Ophthalmol.* 1993 Nov.;21(4):213-7.

[3] O'Mahoney, P. R., Wong, D. T., Ray, J. G. Retinal vein occlusion and traditional risk factors for atherosclerosis. *Arch. Ophthalmol.* 2008 May; 126(5):692-9.

[4] Rehak, J., Rehak, M. Branch retinal vein occlusion: pathogenesis, visual prognosis, and treatment modalities. *Curr. Eye Res.* 2008 Feb.;33(2): 111-31.

[5] Arevalo, J. F., Garcia, R. A., Wu, L., Rodriguez, F. J., Dalma-Weiszhausz, J., Quiroz-Mercado, H., et al. Radial optic neurotomy for central retinal vein occlusion: results of the Pan-American Collaborative Retina Study Group (PACORES). *Retina.* 2008 Oct.;28(8):1044-52.

[6] Dodson, P. M., Galton, D. J., Hamilton, A. M., Blach, R. K. Retinal vein occlusion and the prevalence of lipoprotein abnormalities. *Br. J. Ophthalmol.* 1982 Mar.;66(3):161-4.

[7] Hoh, A. E., Schaal, K. B., Dithmar, S. [Central and branch retinal vein occlusion. Current strategies for treatment in Germany, Austria and Switzerland]. *Ophthalmologe.* 2007 Apr.;104(4):290-4.

[8] Park, C. H., Scott, A. W., Fekrat, S. Effect of oral pentoxifylline on cystoid macular edema associated with central retinal vein occlusion. *Retina.* 2007 Oct.;27(8):1020-5.

[9] Park, D. H., Kim, I. T. Long-term effects of vitrectomy and internal limiting membrane peeling for macular edema secondary to central retinal vein occlusion and hemiretinal vein occlusion. *Retina.* 2010 Jan.; 30(1):117-24.

[10] Argon laser photocoagulation for macular edema in branch vein occlusion. The Branch Vein Occlusion Study Group. *Am. J. Ophthalmol.* 1984 Sep. 15;98(3):271-82.

[11] Evaluation of grid pattern photocoagulation for macular edema in central vein occlusion. The Central Vein Occlusion Study Group M report. *Ophthalmology.* 1995 Oct.;102(10):1425-33.

[12] Ip, M. S., Scott, I. U., VanVeldhuisen, P. C., Oden, N. L., Blodi, B. A., Fisher, M., et al. A randomized trial comparing the efficacy and safety of intravitreal triamcinolone with observation to treat vision loss associated with macular edema secondary to central retinal vein occlusion: the Standard Care vs Corticosteroid for Retinal Vein Occlusion (SCORE) study report 5. *Arch. Ophthalmol.* 2009 Sep.;127(9):1101-14.

[13] Scott, I. U., Ip, M. S., VanVeldhuisen, P. C., Oden, N. L., Blodi, B. A., Fisher, M., et al. A randomized trial comparing the efficacy and safety of intravitreal triamcinolone with standard care to treat vision loss associated with macular Edema secondary to branch retinal vein occlusion: the Standard Care vs Corticosteroid for Retinal Vein Occlusion (SCORE) study report 6. *Arch. Ophthalmol.* 2009 Sep.;127 (9):1115-28.

[14] Haller, J. A., Bandello, F., Belfort, R., Jr., Blumenkranz, M. S., Gillies, M., Heier, J., et al. Dexamethasone intravitreal implant in patients with macular edema related to branch or central retinal vein occlusion twelve-month study results. *Ophthalmology*. 2011 Dec.;118(12):2453-60.

[15] Ramchandran, R. S., Fekrat, S., Stinnett, S. S., Jaffe, G. J. Fluocinolone acetonide sustained drug delivery device for chronic central retinal vein occlusion: 12-month results. *Am. J. Ophthalmol.* 2008 Aug.;146(2):285-91.

[16] Green, W. R., Chan, C. C., Hutchins, G. M., Terry, J. M. Central retinal vein occlusion: a prospective histopathologic study of 29 eyes in 28 cases. 1981. *Retina*. 2005 Jul.-Aug.;25(5 Suppl.):27-55.

[17] Funk, M., Kriechbaum, K., Prager, F., Benesch, T., Georgopoulos, M., Zlabinger, G. J., et al. Intraocular concentrations of growth factors and cytokines in retinal vein occlusion and the effect of therapy with bevacizumab. *Invest. Ophthalmol. Vis. Sci.* 2009 Mar.;50(3):1025-32.

[18] Koss, M. J., Pfister, M., Rothweiler, F., Michaelis, M., Cinatl, J., Schubert, R., et al. Comparison of cytokine levels from undiluted vitreous of untreated patients with retinal vein occlusion. *Acta Ophthalmol.* 2012 Mar.;90(2):e98-e103.

[19] Noma, H., Funatsu, H., Yamasaki, M., Tsukamoto, H., Mimura, T., Sone, T., et al. Aqueous humour levels of cytokines are correlated to vitreous levels and severity of macular oedema in branch retinal vein occlusion. *Eye* (Lond.). 2008 Jan.;22(1):42-8.

[20] Tolentino, M. J., McLeod, D. S., Taomoto, M., Otsuji, T., Adamis, A. P., Lutty, G. A. Pathologic features of vascular endothelial growth

factor-induced retinopathy in the nonhuman primate. *Am. J. Ophthalmol.* 2002 Mar.;133(3):373-85.

[21] Singer, M. A., Cohen, S. R., Groth, S. L., Porbandarwalla, S. Comparing bevacizumab and ranibizumab for initial reduction of central macular thickness in patients with retinal vein occlusions. *Clin. Ophthalmol.* 2013;7:1377-83.

[22] Semenza, G. Signal transduction to hypoxia-inducible factor 1. *Biochem. Pharmacol.* 2002 Sep.;64(5-6):993-8.

[23] Neufeld, G., Cohen, T., Gengrinovitch, S., Poltorak, Z. Vascular endothelial growth factor (VEGF) and its receptors. *FASEB J.* 1999 Jan.; 13(1):9-22.

[24] Ferrara, N., Davis-Smyth, T. The biology of vascular endothelial growth factor. *Endocr. Rev.* 1997 Feb.;18(1):4-25.

[25] Ku, D. D., Zaleski, J. K., Liu, S., Brock, T. A. Vascular endothelial growth factor induces EDRF-dependent relaxation in coronary arteries. *Am. J. Physiol.* 1993 Aug.;265(2 Pt 2):H586-92.

[26] Bates, D. O., Curry, F. E. Vascular endothelial growth factor increases microvascular permeability via a Ca(2+)-dependent pathway. *Am. J. Physiol.* 1997 Aug.;273(2 Pt 2):H687-94.

[27] Roberts, W. G., Palade, G. E. Increased microvascular permeability and endothelial fenestration induced by vascular endothelial growth factor. *J. Cell Sci.* 1995 Jun.;108 ( Pt 6):2369-79.

[28] Dejana, E., Corada, M., Lampugnani, M. G. Endothelial cell-to-cell junctions. *FASEB J.* 1995 Jul.;9(10):910-8.

[29] Wroblewski, J. J., Wells, J. A., 3rd, Adamis, A. P., Buggage, R. R., Cunningham, E. T., Jr., Goldbaum, M., et al. Pegaptanib sodium for macular edema secondary to central retinal vein occlusion. *Arch. Ophthalmol.* 2009 Apr.;127(4):374-8 0.

[30] Wroblewski, J. J., Wells, J. A., 3rd, Gonzales, C. R. Pegaptanib sodium for macular edema secondary to branch retinal vein occlusion. *Am. J. Ophthalmol.* 2010 Jan.;149(1):147-54.

[31] Campochiaro, P. A., Heier, J. S., Feiner, L., Gray, S., Saroj, N., Rundle, A. C., et al. Ranibizumab for macular edema following branch retinal vein occlusion: six-month primary end point results of a phase III study. *Ophthalmology*. 2010 Jun.;117(6):1102-12 e1.

[32] Figueroa, M. S., Ruiz Moreno, J. M. [BRAVO and CRUISE: ranibizumab for the treatment of macular edema secondary to retinal vein occlusion]. *Arch. Soc. Esp. Oftalmol.* 2012 Dec.;87 Suppl. 1:46-53.

[33] Heier, J. S., Campochiaro, P. A., Yau, L., Li, Z., Saroj, N., Rubio, R. G., et al. Ranibizumab for macular edema due to retinal vein occlusions: long-term follow-up in the HORIZON trial. *Ophthalmology*. 2012 Apr.; 119(4):802-9.

[34] Brown, D. M., Campochiaro, P. A., Singh, R. P., Li, Z., Gray, S., Saroj, N., et al. Ranibizumab for macular edema following central retinal vein occlusion: six-month primary end point results of a phase III study. *Ophthalmology*. 2010 Jun.;117(6):1124-33 e1.

[35] Brown, D. M., Heier, J. S., Clark, W. L., Boyer, D. S., Vitti, R., Berliner, A. J., et al. Intravitreal aflibercept injection for macular edema secondary to central retinal vein occlusion: 1-year results from the phase 3 COPERNICUS study. *Am. J. Ophthalmol.* 2013 Mar.;155(3):429-37 e7.

[36] Heier, J. S., Clark, W. L., Boyer, D. S., Brown, D. M., Vitti, R., Berliner, A. J., et al. Intravitreal Aflibercept Injection for Macular Edema Due to Central Retinal Vein Occlusion: Two-Year Results from the COPERNICUS Study. *Ophthalmology*. 2014 Mar. 26.

[37] Korobelnik, J. F., Holz, F. G., Roider, J., Ogura, Y., Simader, C., Schmidt-Erfurth, U., et al. Intravitreal Aflibercept Injection for Macular Edema Resulting from Central Retinal Vein Occlusion: One-Year Results of the Phase 3 GALILEO Study. *Ophthalmology*. 2014 Jan.;121 (1):202-8.

[38] Martin, D. F., Maguire, M. G., Ying, G. S., Grunwald, J. E., Fine, S. L., Jaffe, G. J. Ranibizumab and bevacizumab for neovascular age-related macular degeneration. *N. Engl. J. Med.* 2011 May 19;364(20):1897-908.

[39] Martin, D. F., Maguire, M. G., Fine, S. L., Ying, G. S., Jaffe, G. J., Grunwald, J. E., et al. Ranibizumab and bevacizumab for treatment of neovascular age-related macular degeneration: two-year results. *Ophthalmology*. 2012 Jul.;119(7):1388-98.

[40] Chakravarthy, U., Harding, S. P., Rogers, C. A., Downes, S. M., Lotery, A. J., Wordsworth, S., et al. Ranibizumab versus bevacizumab to treat neovascular age-related macular degeneration: one-year findings from the IVAN randomized trial. *Ophthalmology*. 2012 Jul.;119(7):1399-411.

[41] Krebs, I., Schmetterer, L., Boltz, A., Told, R., Vecsei-Marlovits, V., Egger, S., et al. A randomised double-masked trial comparing the visual outcome after treatment with ranibizumab or bevacizumab in patients with neovascular age-related macular degeneration. *Br. J. Ophthalmol.* 2013 Mar.;97(3):266-71.

[42] Bakri, S. J., Snyder, M. R., Reid, J. M., Pulido, J. S., Ezzat, M. K., Singh, R. J. Pharmacokinetics of intravitreal ranibizumab (Lucentis). *Ophthalmology*. 2007 Dec.;114(12):2179-82.

[43] Wu, L., Martinez-Castellanos, M. A., Quiroz-Mercado, H., Arevalo, J. F., Berrocal, M. H., Farah, M. E., et al. Twelve-month safety of intravitreal injections of bevacizumab (Avastin): results of the Pan-American Collaborative Retina Study Group (PACORES). *Graefes Arch. Clin. Exp. Ophthalmol.* 2008 Jan.;246(1):81-7.

[44] Wu, L., Arevalo, J. F., Roca, J. A., Maia, M., Berrocal, M. H., Rodriguez, F. J., et al. Comparison of two doses of intravitreal bevacizumab (Avastin) for treatment of macular edema secondary to branch retinal vein occlusion: results from the Pan-American Collaborative Retina Study Group at 6 months of follow-up. *Retina.* 2008. Feb.;28(2):212-9.

[45] Hayashi, A., Yunoki, T., Miyakoshi, A., Mitarai, K., Fujino, T., Yanagisawa, S. Intravitreal injection of bevacizumab combined with macular grid laser photocoagulation for macular edema in branch retinal vein occlusion. *Jpn. J. Ophthalmol.* 2011 Nov.;55(6):625-31.

[46] Russo, V., Barone, A., Conte, E., Prascina, F., Stella, A., Noci, N. D. Bevacizumab compared with macular laser grid photocoagulation for cystoid macular edema in branch retinal vein occlusion. *Retina*. 2009 Apr.;29(4):511-5.

[47] Hikichi, T., Higuchi, M., Matsushita, T., Kosaka, S., Matsushita, R., Takami, K., et al. Two-year outcomes of intravitreal bevacizumab therapy for macular oedema secondary to branch retinal vein occlusion. *Br. J. Ophthalmol.* 2014 Feb.;98(2):195-9.

[48] Gokce, G., Sobaci, G., Durukan, A. H., Erdurman, F. C. The comparison of intravitreal triamcinolone and bevacizumab in patients with macular edema secondary to branch retinal vein occlusion. *Clin. Ophthalmol.* 2014;8:355-62.

[49] Yuan, A., Ahmad, B. U., Xu, D., Singh, R. P., Kaiser, P. K., Martin, D. F., et al. Comparison of intravitreal ranibizumab and bevacizumab for the treatment of macular edema secondary to retinal vein occlusion. *Int. J. Ophthalmol.* 2014;7(1):86-91.

[50] Kumagai, K., Ogino, N., Furukawa, M., Larson, E. Three treatments for macular edema because of branch retinal vein occlusion: intravitreous bevacizumab or tissue plasminogen activator, and vitrectomy. *Retina.* 2012 Mar.;32(3):520-9.

[51] Ehrlich, R., Ciulla, T. A., Moss, A. M., Harris, A. Combined treatment of intravitreal bevacizumab and intravitreal triamcinolone in patients with retinal vein occlusion: 6 months of follow-up. *Graefes Arch. Clin. Exp. Ophthalmol.* 2010 Mar.;248(3):375-8 0.

[52] Yilmaz, T., Cordero-Coma, M. Use of bevacizumab for macular edema secondary to branch retinal vein occlusion: a systematic review. *Graefes Arch. Clin. Exp. Ophthalmol.* 2012 Jun.;250(6):787-93.

[53] Ahn, S. J., Ahn, J., Woo, S. J., Park, K. H. Initial dose of three monthly intravitreal injections versus PRN intravitreal injections of bevacizumab for macular edema secondary to branch retinal vein occlusion. *Biomed. Res. Int.* 2013;2013:209735.

[54] Ferrara, D. C., Koizumi, H., Spaide, R. F. Early bevacizumab treatment of central retinal vein occlusion. *Am. J. Ophthalmol.* 2007 Dec.;144 (6): 864-71.

[55] Priglinger, S. G., Wolf, A. H., Kreutzer, T. C., Kook, D., Hofer, A., Strauss, R. W., et al. Intravitreal bevacizumab injections for treatment of central retinal vein occlusion: six-month results of a prospective trial. *Retina*. 2007 Oct.;27(8):1004-12.

[56] Moschos, M. M., Moschos, M. Intraocular bevacizumab for macular edema due to CRVO. A multifocal-ERG and OCT study. *Doc. Ophthalmol.* 2008 Mar.;116(2):147-52.

[57] Epstein, D. L., Algvere, P. V., von Wendt, G., Seregard, S., Kvanta, A. Bevacizumab for macular edema in central retinal vein occlusion: a prospective, randomized, double-masked clinical study. *Ophthalmology*. 2012 Jun.;119(6):1184-9.

[58] Pikkel, J., Chassid, O., Busool, Y., Srour, W., Sharabi-Nov, A., Beiran, I. Bevacizumab for CRVO Associated CME: Effect of Timing and Frequency of Injections on Final Visual Outcome. *J. Ophthalmol.* 2013; 2013:974670.

[59] Huang, P., Niu, W., Ni, Z., Wang, R., Sun, X. A meta-analysis of anti-vascular endothelial growth factor remedy for macular edema secondary to central retinal vein occlusion. *PLoS One*. 2013;8(12):e82454.

[60] Papadopoulou, D. N., Mendrinos, E., Mangioris, G., Donati, G., Pournaras, C. J. Intravitreal ranibizumab may induce retinal arteriolar vasoconstriction in patients with neovascular age-related macular degeneration. *Ophthalmology*. 2009 Sep.;116(9):1755-61.

[61] Spaide, R. F. Peripheral areas of nonperfusion in treated central retinal vein occlusion as imaged by wide-field fluorescein angiography. *Retina*. 2011 May;31(5):829-37.

[62] Manousaridis, K., Talks, J. Macular ischaemia: a contraindication for anti-VEGF treatment in retinal vascular disease? *Br. J. Ophthalmol.* 2012 Feb.;96(2):179-84.

[63] Takahashi, K., Muraoka, K., Kishi, S., Shimizu, K. Formation of retinochoroidal collaterals in central retinal vein occlusion. *Am. J. Ophthalmol.* 1998 Jul.;126(1):91-9.

[64] Gomez-Ulla, F., Abraldes, M. J., Basauri, E., Fernandez, M., Garcia-Layana, A., Gili, P., et al. [SERV clinical practice guidelines: management of retinal vein occlusion. Sociedad Espanola de Retina y Vitreo]. *Arch. Soc. Esp. Oftalmol.* 2010 Sep.;85(9):294-309.

[65] Epstein, D. L., Algvere, P. V., von Wendt, G., Seregard, S., Kvanta, A. Benefit from bevacizumab for macular edema in central retinal vein occlusion: twelve-month results of a prospective, randomized study. *Ophthalmology*. 2012 Dec.;119(12):2587-91.

[66] Campochiaro, P. A., Brown, D. M., Awh, C. C., Lee, S. Y., Gray, S., Saroj, N., et al. Sustained benefits from ranibizumab for macular edema following central retinal vein occlusion: twelve-month outcomes of a phase III study. *Ophthalmology*. 2011 Oct.;118(10):2041-9.

[67] Brown, D. M., Campochiaro, P. A., Bhisitkul, R. B., Ho, A. C., Gray, S., Saroj, N., et al. Sustained benefits from ranibizumab for macular edema following branch retinal vein occlusion: 12-month outcomes of a phase III study. *Ophthalmology*. 2011 Aug.;118(8):1594-602.

[68] Donati, S., Barosi, P., Bianchi, M., Al Oum, M., Azzolini, C. Combined intravitreal bevacizumab and grid laser photocoagulation for macular edema secondary to branch retinal vein occlusion. *Eur. J. Ophthalmol.* 2012 Jul.-Aug.;22(4):607-14.

[69] Hahn, P., Fekrat, S. Best practices for treatment of retinal vein occlusion. *Curr. Opin. Ophthalmol.* 2012 May;23(3):175-81.

In: Macular Edema
Editor: Earl Davison

ISBN: 978-1-63321-584-9


*Chapter 3*

# POSTOPERATIVE CYSTOID MACULAR EDEMA IN DIABETIC PATIENTS: PROPHYLAXIS AND MANAGEMENT

***Javier A. Montero-Moreno*[1,2,*]*, Jose M. Ruiz-Moreno*[3,4]*,***
***Marta Fernandez-Muñoz*[1]*, and María Montero-Sanz*[1]**
[1]Pio del Rio Hortega University Hospital, Valladolid, Spain
[2]Retina Unit, Oftalvist Moncloa, Madrid, Spain
[3]Department of Ophthalmology,
Castilla La Mancha University, Albacete, Spain
[4]Baviera Clinic, European Ophthalmic Institute, Alicante, Spain

## ABSTRACT

The risk of cataracts among diabetic patients is three to five-fold higher than that of healthy population and uneventful phacoemulsification is sometimes associated with an increased risk of aggravation of diabetic retinopathy and macular edema. These increased risks have been related to an over-expression of inflammatory mediators, especially of vascular endothelial growth factor (VEGF). Postoperative macular edema may

* Corresponding author: Javier A. Montero Moreno. Pio Del Rio Hortega University Hospital, Ophthalmology Unit, Calle Dulzaina 2, 47012. Valladolid, Spain. Phone: +34 983 420 400. Fax: +34 983 215 365. E-mail: javiermonmor@gmail.com.

resolve spontaneously, but most frequently it will reduce the expected visual acuity improvement. Among the most usual strategies for the prevention of postoperative macular edema in diabetic patients, preoperative laser photocoagulation and intra operative intravitreal steroids and anti-VEGF drugs have been advocated. Similarly, it has been suggested that topical anti-inflammatory drops may improve visual outcome after surgery. Nd-YAG laser treatment of postoperative posterior capsular opacification can also be linked to an increased risk of macular edema. Spectral Domain Optical Coherence Tomography is a very sensitive tool for the identification of macular changes associated with surgery.

In this chapter we revise the most usual strategies for the prophylaxis and management of postoperative macular edema in diabetic patients as well as our experience and the results of the most recent clinical trials.

## INTRODUCTION

Diabetes mellitus (DM) is one of the fastest growing epidemics worldwide and is estimated to affect 300 million people by year 2025 [1]. Cataracts are a frequent cause of decreased visual acuity (VA) among diabetics. Cortical and posterior sub capsular cataracts are more frequent and appear earlier in diabetics, and DM is considered the third most frequent risk factor for the crystalline lens opacification after age and genetics, leading to decreased VA and increased difficulty for the follow-up of diabetic retinopathy (DR). The incidence of cataract surgery among diabetic patients is three to five-fold higher than that of healthy population, and the risk of cataracts increases in aged patients, females and in patients with proteinuria [1].

Both cataracts and diabetic macular edema (DME) are common causes of decreased VA among diabetic patients. Laser photocoagulation is a well-known treatment for DME; however, effective laser treatment may not be possible in diabetic patients with significant crystalline lens opacifications. As long as the cataract density permits it, laser treatment of DME should precede phacoemulsification surgery and cataract removal be delayed until the macular edema subsides.

The dilemma in this situation is that cataracts significantly reduce the view of the fundus, limiting the efficacy and safety of macular laser photocoagulation. Therefore, other treatment options such as the intravitreal injection of pharmacologic agents have been used in these patients, before, during, or after cataract surgery.

Cataract surgery in patients with non proliferative diabetic retinopathy (NPDR) has been traditionally associated with progression of the retinopathy defined as the appearance of a clinically significant macular edema (CSME), increased intra retinal hemorrhages and hard exudates or progression to proliferative diabetic retinopathy (PDR). Even uneventful phacoemulsification has been associated with increased DME in diabetic patients [2-4].

Yet, it is still unclear whether DME worsening is caused by the surgery itself, or is just simply the natural progression of the disease. Some authors advise performing early phacoemulsification in diabetic patients with cataracts in order to achieve optimal posterior pole visualization clearing the ambiguity of the cause of decreased vision. According to their findings, uncomplicated phacoemulsification does not accelerate DME or DR, provided that glycemic control and co-morbids are well addressed [5].

Pollack et al. showed that 81% of patients with preoperative NPDR will develop a cystoid macular edema (CME) after cataract surgery vs. 32% of patients without DR [6].

During the past 15 years optical coherence tomography (OCT) has become an indispensable diagnostic tool providing high resolution, cross sectional, in vivo images of the retina and the choroid, supplementing the result of ophthalmoscopy, fluorescein angiography (FA) and ultrasound examination with a quantitative measurement that allows us to assess the progression of the disease and the therapeutic success.

Evaluation of the postoperative macular edema (ME) requires a proper identification of the real cause of the edema, whether it is secondary to the surgery itself (as in the case of the Irvine-Gass syndrome) or is related to DR.

Postoperative CME is recognized as a cause of suboptimal postoperative visual outcome. The diagnosis of CME and DME can generally be made on slit lamp biomicroscopy with evidence of perifoveal cystic spaces and be confirmed with FA and OCT.

Early optic disk hyper fluorescence associated with early fluorescein leakage from the perifoveal capillary bed and a late petaloid frame are highly suggestive of an Irvine-Gass syndrome and therefore, a trend towards self-resolution. The incidence of CME is in the range of 1-2% using modern phacoemulsification techniques [7].

Fluid leak from perifoveal vessels is induced by inflammatory mediators, resulting in intraretinal fluid accumulation and decreased retinal function, and is generally associated with rupture of the posterior capsule, vitreous loss, iris incarceration or use of iris-fixated lenses [7]. Most of the authors recommend waiting for self-resolution of postoperative ME during at least 6 months.

Dowler et al. described the natural history of ME after cataract surgery in diabetic eyes before OCT became available, by means of a prospective clinical and angiographic trial on 32 patients with diabetes undergoing cataract surgery. In the first postoperative year, macular hyper fluorescence increased in 30 of 32 eyes, returning to its preoperative level within 1 year of surgery in 13 eyes. Similarly, optic diskc hyper fluorescence increased in 27 eyes, returning to its preoperative level within 1 year of surgery in 19 eyes.

Clinically significant DME was identified in 18 eyes during the first year and did not resolve spontaneously within 1 year of the surgical procedure in any of the 5 eyes in which it had been present at the time of surgery; and resolved in 9 of 13 eyes in which it arose within the first 6 months after surgery. In this series, preoperative CSME was associated with poorer VA one year after surgery [8].

The occurrence of postoperative ME in diabetic patients is controversial. Some studies suggest that DME after cataract surgery occurs predominantly in people with concurrent preexisting significant DME, while other reports indicate that preexisting DME is not required for postoperative DME [3].

The Diabetic Retinopathy Clinical Research Network (DRCR.net) performed a non-interventional study to assess the incidence of central-involving ME as defined by OCT after cataract surgery [9]. In this multicenter, prospective, observational study, 293 eyes with DR and without definite DME defined by OCT underwent cataract surgery. The median age was 65 years with a median VA letter score of 69 letters. 44% of eyes had been previously treated for DME. The authors concluded that the risk of developing central DME increased in eyes with DR and central sparing DME immediately prior to surgery. However, DME may also appear after cataract surgery in diabetic patients without DR, as was shown by Katsimpris et al. [10].

These authors evaluated 98 patients (49 with type 2 diabetes with no DR and 49 healthy controls) before cataract surgery and 1, 3, 6, and 12 months postoperatively. Even though preoperative OCT showed no significant difference between both groups, postoperative foveal thickness significantly increased in diabetics at all time-points of the follow-up period when compared to controls with a 7-fold incidence of CME.

Jaffe et al. reported a small series of diabetic patients with symmetric NPDR who were operated on by extra capsular surgery with intraocular lens (IOL) implantation and followed during an average 18 months. Nineteen patients presented bilateral progression of DR, defined as the appearance of CSME, an increase in intra retinal hemorrhages or hard exudates, or the development of PDR.

Cataract surgery was followed by asymmetric progression of NPDR that was more pronounced in the operated eye; none of these patients presented progression of NPDR in the fellow eye alone [11].

Ostri et al. [12] assessed visual acuity outcomes after phacoemulsification in a cohort study between 1999 and 2008 on a large population of 7 323 diabetic patients with all degrees of DR. Corrected distance VA increased significantly after cataract surgery in all diabetic retinopathy categories, and visual gain correlated positively with preoperative VA and negatively with the degree of DR and age. Patients with previous focal laser treatment for CSME had a higher risk for not improving after cataract surgery.

Yet, there is no complete evidence that cataract surgery causes progression of DR or DME, especially among those patients with low-risk DR, and it has been suggested that worse visual outcomes are correlated with more severe retinopathy [3] and poorer glycemic control [13].

According to other series diabetes does not significantly influence thickening of the macular regions after uncomplicated cataract surgery, even though non-significant thickening of the perifoveal area may occur. Biro et al. performed a prospective study using OCT in 18 eyes of 18 diabetic patients who underwent uneventful cataract surgery in order to evaluate the changes of the foveal and perifoveal area [14].

Data were collected one day before the operation, and at days 1, 7, 30, and 60, using fellow eyes as controls. According to their findings, no significant thickness changes were observed at day 1; however, a significant increase in macular thickness was detected on the postoperative 7, 30, and 60 days.

Eriksson et al. [15] performed a prospective study in order to assess the appearance of CME impairing visual recovery as complication of cataract surgery. They compared 34 patients with type-2 diabetes and moderate DR with no previous DME, and 35 controls by means of FA and OCT. VA was measured preoperatively, and after surgery at day 7, week 6 and month 6. The authors observed no statistically significant differences in VA before surgery, at day 7 or at 6 months.

There was a significant difference at 6 weeks with lower VA in the diabetic group, and 6% of control and 12% of diabetic eyes developed a CSME between day 7 and week 6. FA leakage occurred in 23% of control eyes vs. 76% of diabetic eyes, with similar changes on OCT and with poor correlation between VA and retinal thickening.

Hykin et al. reported on 56 eyes with PDR that presented progression of PDR after cataract surgery, with iris neovascularization, worsening of CSME, uveitis, vitritis or vitreous hemorrhage [16].

The authors recommended cataract surgery only in those patients in whom cataract progression prevented management of DR in order to achieve stabilization of DR and not in order to improve VA.

## PATHOGENESIS

The main causes of poor VA outcome after uneventful cataract surgery in diabetic patients are complications of fibrovascular proliferation and DME. The severity of DME and DR, and the increased vitreous concentration of pro-inflammatory factors associated with surgery may jeopardize the result of cataract surgery. OCT is a very useful tool due to its capability to determine macular thickness with great reproducibility, as well as identifying epiretinal membranes and vitreoretinal tractions.

The main regulator of physiological and pathological angiogenesis in the eye is vascular endothelial growth factor (VEGF). Several isoforms of VEGF have been identified that derive from the same gene family, and among them VEGFA seems to be related to vascular proliferation.

Among the effects of VEGF in the retina, endothelial migration and proliferation have been associated with formation of micro aneurysms and neovascularization, and VEGF-induced hyper permeability causes CSME by disruption of the *zonula occludens*, induction of endothelial fenestration and fragmentation of the endothelium.

On the other side, VEGF plays a neuroprotective role on the glia, retinal pigment epithelium (RPE) and retinal neurons. The expression and vitreous and aqueous concentrations of VEGF increase under hypoxic and inflammatory conditions such as DR and retinal vein occlusion, and in lower concentrations in exudative age related macular degeneration (AMD) and myopic choroidal neovascularization.

DME is believed to be secondary to multiple biochemical and cellular changes that eventually lead to leakage and exudation. Factors involved in increased retinal vascular permeability are interleukin-6 and VEGF as well as an impaired blood–retina barrier [17]. Aqueous levels of VEGF and interleukin-6 are over-expressed after cataract surgery [18] and significantly correlate with postoperative worsening of ME in diabetic eyes [19].

Hartnett et al. [20] studied associations between serum and aqueous VEGF levels and between insulin-like growth factor 1 (IGF-1) and ME after phacoemulsification in diabetic patients. They performed a prospective study on 36 consecutive diabetic patients undergoing planned phacoemulsification.

Four patients with CSME were preoperatively treated by focal laser photocoagulation. Aqueous and blood samples for VEGF and IGF-1 were taken preoperatively. Mean aqueous VEGF levels showed a direct correlation with the severity of retinopathy and were higher in patients with preoperative CSME. One month after surgery aqueous VEGF levels correlated significantly with clinical changes in central macular thickness (CMT) in diabetic patients.

VEGF inhibition induces retinal arteriolar vasoconstriction; reduced blood flow in an already compromised tissue may lead to irreversible changes in the retina. Intravitreal anti VEGF drugs may also reduce fenestration of the endothelium of the choriocapillaris; therefore, it has been suggested that the effect of these drugs may further reduce oxygenation of the ischemic retina. However, it has been observed that VEGF blockade reduces retinal non perfusion, and may have a positive effect in the reduction of retinal ischemia in DR [21]. Bevacizumab and ranibizumab induce a non-selective blockade of all VEGF isoforms and are frequently used in the treatment of DME, reducing macular thickness and improving visual acuity, even though their use after repeated injections may eventually increase retinal apoptosis and capillary dropout.

## PREOPERATIVE CARE

The preoperative work-up of a diabetic patient with cataracts must include certain data such as the type, duration and quality of control of glycaemia, preferably including glycosilated hemoglobin and other systemic factors such as hypercholesterolemia, arterial hypertension, renal or hepatic insufficiency;, and ocular history such as previous laser treatment and surgery, presence of DME or neovascular glaucoma, and previous cataract surgery and its outcome in the fellow eye. Ocular examination must evaluate the presence or absence of iris neovascularization, gonioscopy, and dilated funduscopy and FA in order to ascertain the presence and amount of DME and ischemia.

FA is especially indicated in eyes that have not been previously treated by pan retinal laser and whenever ME or ischemia are suspected in order to perform laser or pharmacological treatment before surgery, when possible. Postoperative progression of DR has been related to the staging of DR at the time of surgery, glycaemia control and the duration of DR.

The Royal College of Ophthalmologists (Table 1) [22] and the Spanish Retina and Vitreous Society (Table 2) [23] have published their guidelines for the management of ME, where they recommend to delay cataract surgery as long as fundus visualization and laser treatment is possible, and phacoemulsification will only be indicated when these limits are exceeded.

The patient must be carefully monitored during at least 6 months after surgery and laser treatment be performed if required in case the surgical trauma induces progression of DR.

Presently, improved control of diabetes, better surgical techniques with in-bag IOL implantation as well as improved management of DR have improved the visual outcome of diabetic patients with cataracts. Phacoemulsification has reduced postoperative complications, and an adequate management of DR and patient selection have improved VA outcome in diabetic patients.

## MANAGEMENT

It has been reported that cataract surgery may induce an increased macular thickness during the first three months after surgery that in some cases will be self resolved [24]. Preexisting DME should be managed in advance to cataract surgery if the media are transparent enough. Otherwise, preoperative anti-VEGF or steroid treatment can be performed.

**Table 1. The Royal College of Ophthalmologists guidelines on the management of cataract surgery in patients with diabetic macular edema [22]**

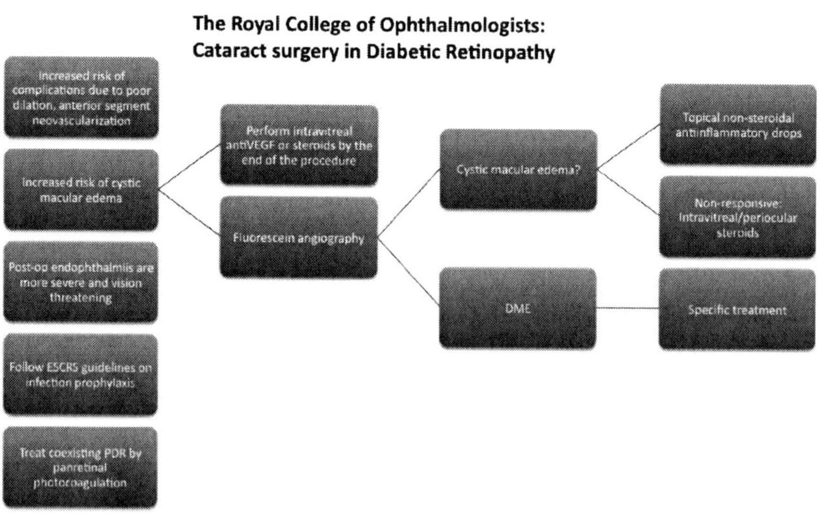

**Table 2. The Spanish Retina and Vitreous Society guidelines on the management of cataract surgery in patients with diabetic macular edema [23]**

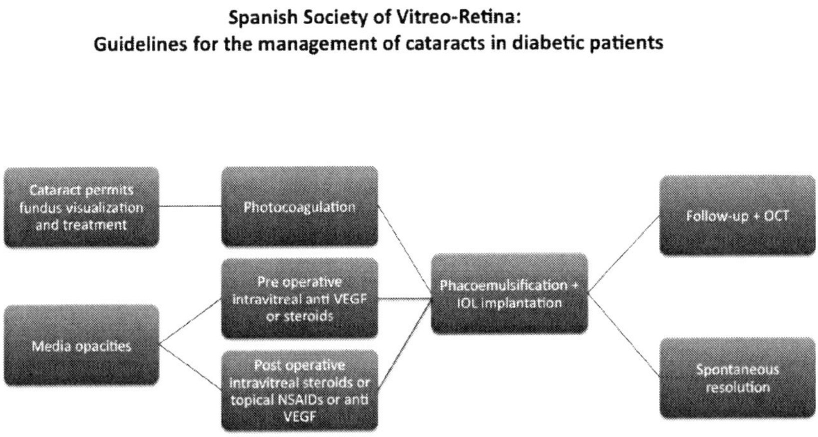


Several small series have been reported on this subject and a few randomized clinical trials have been performed or are under way.

Unfortunately, results from these clinical trials have not been released, even after completion of the studies [25-27]. Several modalities such as non-steroidal anti-inflammatory agents, carbonic anhydrase inhibitors, corticosteroids, hyperbaric oxygen, laser photocoagulation and vitrectomy with internal limiting membrane peeling have been tried with varied success for the management of inflammatory CME.

Several authors have tried to improve functional and anatomic outcomes of DME by means of grid laser photocoagulation of the macula as well as intravitreal steroids and anti VEGF drugs. Steroids reduce intraocular inflammation, cell proliferation, and neovascularization, therefore reducing the expression of vascular growth factors and improving the integrity of the blood–retinal barrier. However, among their well-known side effects, steroid-induced glaucoma is frequently a serious adverse event that may be difficult to treat [28]. Intravitreal anti VEGF therapy has also been evaluated in the literature. Pegaptanib sodium has been reported to improve DME when administered every 6 weeks for 12 weeks to 30 weeks [29]. More recently several series have been reported using bevacizumab [30-32], ranibizumab [33, 34] and aflibercept in the management of DME [35].

LASER TREATMENT: Preoperative laser may improve visual outcome as was proved in the Early Treatment Diabetic Retinopathy Study (ETDRS) [1]; in this series, VA outcome was better among patients who had been previously treated by argon laser compared with other series of untreated patients. Among the eyes from the ETDRS, there were 270 eyes that underwent cataract surgery; 81% of them had been previously treated by photocoagulation before surgery. One year after surgery VA gain greater than 2 lines occurred in 64% of the operated-on eyes treated by early photocoagulation (46% of eyes achieved visual acuity better than 70 ETDRS letters) vs. 59% of eyes assigned to deferral of photocoagulation (36% achieved visual acuity better than 70 letters) after surgery, with little change in VA between 1 and 2 years postoperatively. Lens surgery was associated with a borderline statistically significant increased risk of progression of DR. These VA results were better than the results published for similar patients and were attributed to a more intensive photocoagulation of DR lesions [1].

On this basis, photocoagulation is recommended before cataract surgery for patients with severe PDR or CSME.

Suto et al. evaluated the outcomes in 29 patients with DR and cataract that had pan retinal photocoagulation (PRP) first and cataract surgery second in one eye and cataract surgery followed by PRP in the fellow eye. VA $\geq$70 letters was statistically significantly more frequent in the surgery-first group (97%) than in the PRP-first group (69%) ($p = 0.012$), with a lower rate of progression of DME in the surgery-first group [36]. Aqueous flare intensities measured as an indicator of intraocular inflammation were significantly higher in the PRP-first group and they that persisted until 3 months after surgery.

Generally speaking, DR should be treated in advance prior to cataract surgery, especially when associated to signs of risk of PDR. DME should be treated in advance to cataract surgery and be re-evaluated three months later.

Intraocular neovascularization should be treated in advance to cataract surgery and the surgical procedure be postponed until the new vessels have regressed.

ADJUVANT DRUGS: Pharmacological treatment is very useful in the management of DR, combining phacoemulsification with the intravitreal injection of steroids or anti-VEGF drugs, permitting a reduction of ME and laser treatment in the immediate postoperative period.

Even though the precise pathogenic mechanism of diffuse ME in DR still remains unknown, it is mediated by a breakdown of the blood-retinal barrier, especially located at the micro aneurysms with increased permeability, intraretinal microvascular anomalies and dilated retinal capillaries.

Hyperglycemia induces retinal hypoxia and increases VEGF expression. Other mediators such as prostaglandins and pigment-derived growth factor (PDGF) seem to play a similar role. Previous studies have evaluated the use of intravitreal injections in the same session with phacoemulsification surgery in patients with diabetes with both DME and lens opacities.

## Intravitreal Implant of Dexamethasone

In search for the ideal corticosteroid preparation, a Dexamethasone Posterior Segment Drug Delivery System (Dexamethasone DDS - Ozurdex®, Allergan Inc, Irvine, California) was recently developed. This is a sustained release intravitreal implant containing 700μg dexamethasone that has been approved by the United States Food and Drug Administration (FDA) and the European Drug Agency (EMEA). Promising results have been shown in certain patients with persistent DME receiving this intravitreal drug delivery system with improvement in VA. Ram et al. reported on two anecdotic cases of inadvertent injection of dexamethasone implant into the capsular bag of two eyes of two diabetic patients DME. The accident was followed by successful completion of phacoemulsification and IOL implantation, without recurrences of ME at 1 year follow-up [37].

A clinical trial is presently under way recruiting patients in order to determine the effect of intravitreal long acting dexamethasone implant in improving anatomic and functional outcomes of cataract surgery in patients with DME [27]. This study introduces a novel concept of using intraoperative Ozurdex® implant in patients with DM while undergoing cataract surgery to minimize the worsening of diabetic maculopathy. The study will randomize patients to be treated by conventional phacoemulsification with IOL implantation or phacoemulsification with IOL implantation and intraoperative intravitreal injection of a dexamethasone drug delivery system.

## Intravitreal Triamcinolone Acetonide

The precise mechanism of steroids in the management of DME is unknown, though it is generally accepted that they are non-specific suppressors of inflammation inhibiting the arachidonic cascade, reducing the production of prostaglandins and the expression of VEGF.

Other reported effects of intravitreal TA steroids are the inhibition of the blood-retinal barrier breakdown and its anti proliferative effect.

Triamcinolone acetonide (TA) (TA) has been widely used as periocular and intravitreal adjuvant. TA is a long acting depot steroid. It is commercially available as a cheap, sterile, hydrophobic suspension in benzyl alcohol. Intravitreal injection of TA has been associated with various complications, of which cataracts, endophthalmitis and increased intraocular pressure (IOP) are among the most significant [38].

In 2008 Kim et al. assessed the effect of a single intraoperative sub-Tenon injection of TA on the progression of CME after cataract surgery in a prospective controlled study involving 46 eyes of 23 diabetic patients. One month after surgery VA showed a greater improvement in the TA group and the incidence of CME was higher in the control group, even though TA did not affect DR progression over the 6-month follow-up [39].

Habib et al. evaluated the safety and effectivity of intravitreal TA combined with cataract surgery in patients with DME. They evaluated 18 eyes from12 patients, including eyes with persistent DME unresponsive to laser treatment and eyes with no adequate preoperative view for laser treatment. Postoperatively, 15 eyes had completely dry fovea at 2 weeks, with significant VA gain [40]. The effect of peroperative intravitreal TA was evaluated by Ahmadabadi et al. in a prospective randomized controlled study on 41 eyes [41]. There was no statistically significant difference between both groups in VA at any follow-up examination, even though CMT was significantly lower in the treatment group.

The authors concluded that intravitreal TA had no effect on VA gain.

Beer et al. reported a great variability of the intraocular concentration of TA among the different subjects after a single intraocular injection of 4mg TA. Measurable concentrations of TA were observed during approximately 3 months in non-vitrectomized eyes with a mean half-life of 18.6 days in non-vitrectomized patients vs. less than 3.2 days in vitrectomized eyes [42].

Lam et al. assessed the efficacy of phacoemulsification combined with intravitreal 4mg TA injection in 19 patients with DME. Patients were observed until 6 months postoperatively. Eleven eyes showed VA gain ≥2 lines; mean CMT decreased from 449μm to 321μm at 2 months. The authors concluded that the combination of phacoemulsification with intravitreal 4mg TA was safe and effective in diabetic patients with cataract and ME [43].

The largest trial on the effects of intravitreal TA compared two different doses (1mg and 4mg) with focal/grid photocoagulation for the treatment of

DME on 840 eyes [44]. Mean VA at 4 months was better in the 4mg TA group.

One year after the procedure there were no significant differences among groups in mean VA. During the second year mean VA was better in the laser group than in the other two groups. OCT generally showed an inverse correlation with VA results. IOP showed an increase in 16% to 33% of eyes treated with intravitreal TA.

We have performed a retrospective study on 25 eyes from 25 patients with DM who underwent cataract surgery combined with intravitreal injection of 4mg TA. Mean age at baseline was 74±9 years and 14 of them were females. The average (known) duration of diabetes prior to surgery was 15±9 years, and the mean preoperative VA was 58.1±9.5 ETDRS letters. Mean CMT as determined by SD-OCT was 337±77μm.

One month after uneventful phacoemulsification with Acrysof SN60WF IOL implantation (Alcon, Fort Worth, TX), and intravitreal injection of 4mg TA followed by topical dexamethasone and tobramycine, mean CMT was 290±97μm, and by month three after surgery it was 352±113μm, with an average VA change of 5.9 ETDRS letters. However there was marked inter individual variability with patients that presented mild extrafoveal edema with good and stable response to intravitreal TA (Figure 1), patients with early response to TA who presented ME recurrences by month 3 (Figure 2) and patients with no response to TA who presented a progressive retinal thickening despite successive intravitreal injections of TA (Figure 3). Two patients developed transient increased IOP that required pharmacological treatment.

Our findings suggest that intravitreal TA combined with cataract surgery may help reducing retinal thickness after uneventful phacoemulsification in diabetic patients with DME. However their effects are transient and with great inter individual variability and usually require further injections.

## Intravitreal Ranibizumab

Ranibizumab (Lucentis®, Hoffmann-La RocheGenentech, Novartis) is an anti-VEGF agent formed by a modified Fab fraction of a humanized monoclonal antibody that was initially tried for exudative AMD and was later successfully tried to treat ME in patients with diabetic retinopathy and retinal vein occlusion (RVO). Ranibizumab shows a high affinity for VEGFA. The intravitreal use of ranibizumab (IVR) combined with phacoemulsification has been reported with varied anatomical and functional success.

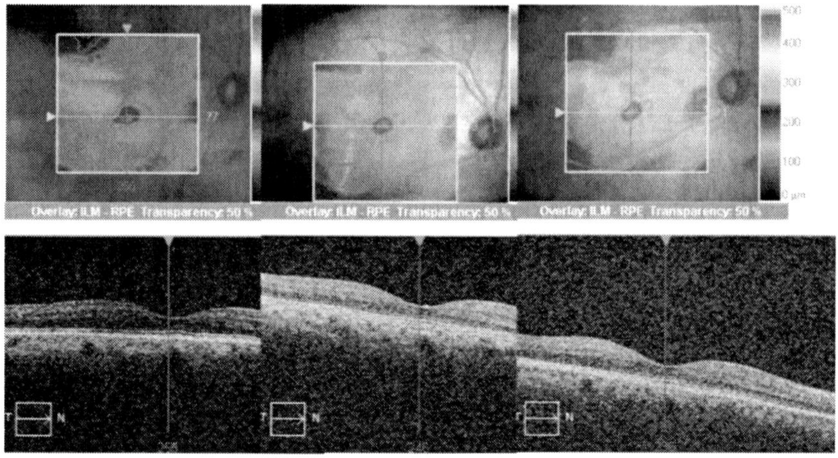


Figure 1. Preoperative (left) and postoperative Optical Coherence Tomography at 1 month (center) and 3 months (right) of one patient with NPDR treated by intravitreal triamcinolone simultaneous to uneventful phacoemulsification. Central macular thickness remains stable after surgery.

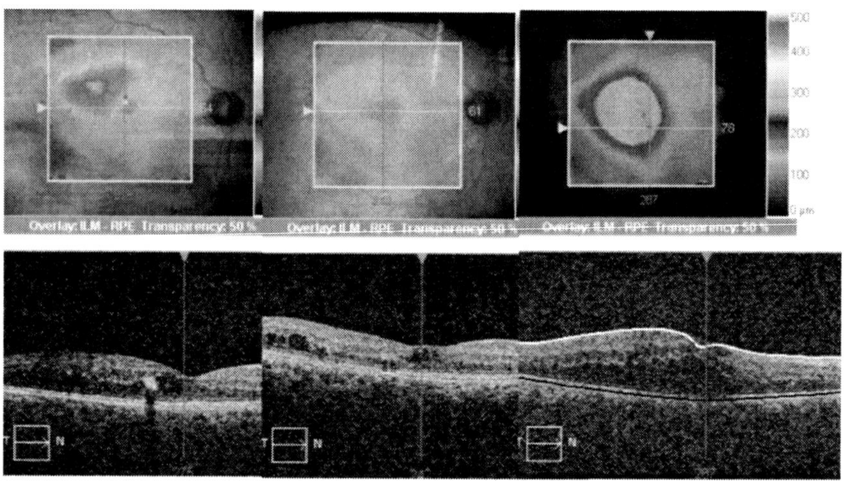


Figure 2. Preoperative (left) and postoperative Optical Coherence Tomography at 1 month (center) and 3 months (right) of one patient with NPDR treated by intravitreal triamcinolone simultaneous to uneventful phacoemulsification. Preoperative non-central DME initially responds to intravitreal triamcinolone (center) and reappears three months after surgery as the vitreous drug levels drop.

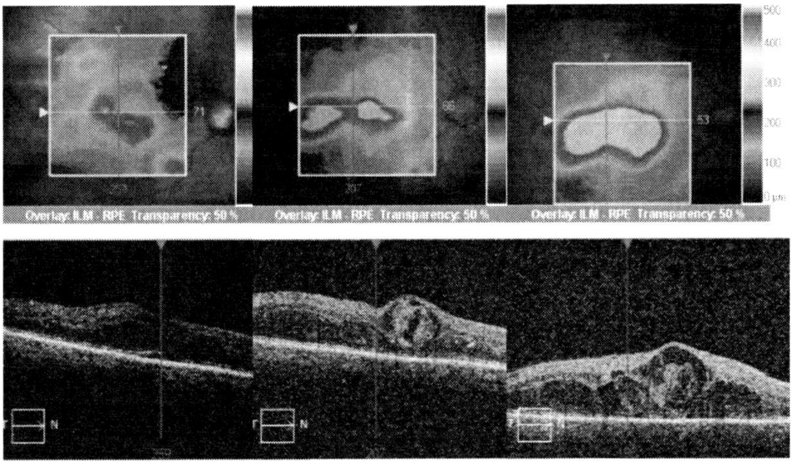

Figure 3. Preoperative (left) and postoperative Optical Coherence Tomography at 1 month (center) and 3 months (right) of one patient with NPDR treated by intravitreal triamcinolone simultaneous to uneventful phacoemulsification. Preoperative central DME does not respond to intravitreal triamcinolone (center) and CMT shows a progressive increase after surgery with large intraretinal cysts.

In order to investigate CMT and VA changes after one 0.5mg IVR during phacoemulsification in eyes with DME refractory to laser treatment, Rauen et al. performed a prospective study on 11 eyes with DME refractory to laser therapy that were treated by phacoemulsification combined with IVR [45].

Patients were evaluated preoperatively and at 1, 4, 8, and 12 weeks postoperatively. Mean CMT was 400±30μm at baseline and did not change significantly at any postoperative study visit ($p > 0.05$). Mean VA was 37±78 ETDRS letters at baseline and was significantly improved at weeks 1 (67±77), 4 (66±80), 8 (68 ± 81), and 12 (63±79) after treatment ($p < 0.05$), and this VA gain was attributed to cataract removal.

A prospective randomized clinical trial evaluated the effectiveness of IVR combined with cataract surgery for the prevention of CSME in patients with DR [46]. This study included 54 eyes with a previous diagnosis of NPDR without ME preoperatively that were randomized to receive an intraoperative IVR or sham injection, associated with standardized phacoemulsification surgery. One month after surgery the incidence of CSME was 26% and 4% in the control group and in the treatment group respectively, and at three months it was 22% and 4%, respectively, suggesting that IVR immediately after phacoemulsification prevents CSME in patients with NPDR.

## Intravitreal Bevacizumab

Bevacizumab (Avastin®, Hoffmann-La Roche) is a full-length humanized monoclonal antibody that binds all forms of VEGFA, and was primarily indicated and approved to be used systemically to treat metastasized cancers, even though due to its lower price when used intravitreously compared to other intravitreous drugs and its availability, it has been used extensively off-label to treat retinal neovascular and edematous conditions secondary to DR, retinal venous occlusion and choroidal neovascularization. The effects of intravitreal bevacizumab (IVB) on neovascular AMD have been compared with those of IVR in randomized prospective masked controlled clinical trials and found to be similar and non-inferior.

However, despite its widespread use in other conditions, its efficacy has not been evaluated in DME with such criteria.

Akinci et al. retrospectively revised the records of 31 patients with CSME and cataract, who had been operated on by uneventful phacoemulsification with IVB, followed by focal or modified grid laser photocoagulation 1 month after the surgery. In their series, mean VA improved from 35±20 ETDRS letters preoperatively to 68±45 letters and 71±40 at months 1 and 3 after surgery, respectively ($p=0.004$). These visual changes were associated with similar reduction of CMT as determined by OCT from 387.5 ± 109.5µm to 292.7 ± 57.2 and 275.5 ± 40.3 respectively ($p < 0.001$, $p < 0.001$).

Cheema et al. performed a prospective study in which they recruited 68 patients with DME undergoing cataract surgery that were randomized to be treated by conventional phacoemulsification or combined surgery with intra operative IVB, observing that there was no difference in terms of VA or CMT, even though they noticed lower rates of DR progression in the treated group six months after surgery.

Wahab et al. prospectively evaluated 38 diabetic patients with poor preoperative glycaemia control (HbAlc level 8.36±1.93, range 6.3 - 12.3) who had been treated by macular grid treatment and were operated on by phacoemulsification and intra operative IVB. Mean preoperative duration of diabetes was 9.92±5.5 years. Six months after surgery corrected VA was 85 to 60 ETDRS letters in 23 eyes, 70 letters in 11 eyes and 55 letters in 4 eyes, concluding that prior macular grid laser and intra operative IVB is a safe combined therapy in DM patients undergoing cataract surgery [47].

Lanzagorta-Aresti et al. randomized 26 patients with moderate NPDR and diffuse DME to be treated by IVB vs. saline injection immediately after cataract surgery [48].

VA was significantly better in the treated group during the following 6 months, and correlated with no significant increase of CMT within the treated group, suggesting the positive effect of IVB in DM cataract surgery.

In a similar way, Takamura et al. performed a prospective, randomized, cohort study on 42 eyes with DME, treated either by cataract surgery only or combined with 1.25mg IVB. The authors found no preoperative significant differences in CMT, VA or systemic condition between both groups.

After surgery the IVB group showed a significant improvement in retinal thickness with significantly better visual results than the control group, with significant relationship between CMT and VA in both groups that lasted at least three months [49].

Chen et al. retrospectively evaluated 29 eyes operated on by phacoemulsification; 15 of them had been treated by IVB after cataract surgery. Three months after surgery both groups had improved VA and the IVB group showed a significant reduction in central macular thickness [50].

Unfortunately the small samples evaluated in all these studies as well as the varied inclusion criteria, their non-prospective nature and the short follow-up are limitations to draw conclusions.

These results suggest that certain benefit can be achieved from adjunctive treatment at the time of phacoemulsification, especially in eyes with no preoperative retinal thickening. Intravitreal drugs seem to be less effective to treat pre-existing DME when associated with cataract surgery.

## Topical Anti-Inflammatory Drugs

Topical medical treatment of DR has not been successful to date. Kern et al. assessed the effect of topical nepafenac (an anti-inflammatory drug that may reach therapeutic concentration in the retina after topical administration) administered during the early stages of DR in an animal model of streptozotocin-induced diabetic rats. Increased levels of retinal prostaglandin E(2), superoxide, cyclooxygenase-2, and retinal micro vessels leukostasis were significantly inhibited by nepafenac, though no changes on VEGF and nitric oxide (NO) were observed. Topical nepafenac achieved sufficient drug delivery to the retina and changes in retinal vascular metabolism, function, and morphology were inhibited, with little or no effect on diabetes-induced retinal ganglion cell deaths [51]. Wolf et al. retrospectively compared the incidence of visually significant ME after uneventful phacoemulsification on 240 patients treated with topical prednisolone vs. 210 patients treated with topical prednisolone and nepafenac 0.1%. Both groups were clinically comparable in sex distribution, history of diabetes, hypertension or cardiac disease and all patients were followed for at least 1 month postoperatively. After observing visually significant pseudophakic ME in 5 patients treated with prednisolone alone and in none of the patients treated with prednisolone and nepafenac the authors concluded that topical prednisolone alone might be associated to a significantly higher incidence of visually significant pseudophakic ME than those treated with combined treatment with nepafenac [52].

The appropriate management of diabetic patients undergoing cataract surgery is still unclear. Even though older studies suggested that cataract surgery caused progression of diabetic retinal disease, more recent phacoemulsification surgery does not support this conclusion and the question remains open whether progression of DME and DR is a result of surgical trauma or just reflects a natural progression of the disease.

Small-scale studies on adjuvant steroidal or anti-VEGF agents performed at the time of cataract surgery suggest improved outcomes in terms of VA and ME as well as progression of DR, especially among those patients with poorly controlled or refractory ME.

Future larger, prospective, controlled trials with longer follow-up will help further elucidate the real effect of these treatments on cataract surgery outcomes, providing more information on the risks and benefits of their association. It is likely that a longer delay is needed between PRP and cataract surgery. The usually good visual outcomes after phacoemulsification highlight the importance of proper preoperative management of macular edema.

## REFERENCES


[1] Chew, E. Y., Benson, W. E., Remaley, N. A., Lindley, A. A., Burton, T. C., Csaky, K., et al. Results after lens extraction in patients with diabetic retinopathy: early treatment diabetic retinopathy study report number 25. *Arch. Ophthalmol.* 1999 Dec.;117(12):1600-6.

[2] Degenring, R. F., Vey, S., Kamppeter, B., Budde, W. M., Jonas, J. B., Sauder, G. Effect of uncomplicated phacoemulsification on the central retina in diabetic and non-diabetic subjects. *Graefes Arch. Clin. Exp. Ophthalmol.* 2007 Jan.;245(1):18-23.

[3] Kim, S. J., Equi, R., Bressler, N. M. Analysis of macular edema after cataract surgery in patients with diabetes using optical coherence tomography. *Ophthalmology.* 2007 May;114(5):881-9.

[4] Romero-Aroca, P., Fernandez-Ballart, J., Almena-Garcia, M., Mendez-Marin, I., Salvat-Serra, M., Buil-Calvo, J. A. Nonproliferative diabetic retinopathy and macular edema progression after phacoemulsification: prospective study. *J. Cataract Refract. Surg.* 2006 Sep.;32(9):1438-44.

[5] Wahab, S., Faiz-ur-Rab, K., Das Hargun, L. Early phacoemulsification in diabetic cataract for early recognition and management of diabetic macular oedema. *J. Coll. Physicians Surg. Pak.* 2013 Jun.;23(6):401-4.

[6] Pollack, A., Leiba, H., Bukelman, A., Oliver, M. Cystoid macular oedema following cataract extraction in patients with diabetes. *Br. J. Ophthalmol.* 1992 Apr.;76(4):221-4.

[7] Ray, S., D'Amico, D. J. Pseudophakic cystoid macular edema. *Semin. Ophthalmol.* 2002 Sep.-Dec.;17(3-4):167-80.

[8] Dowler, J. G., Sehmi, K. S., Hykin, P. G., Hamilton, A. M. The natural history of macular edema after cataract surgery in diabetes. *Ophthalmology.* 1999 Apr.;106(4):663-8.

[9] Macular Edema After Cataract Surgery in Eyes Without Preoperative Central-Involved Diabetic Macular Edema. *JAMA Ophthalmol.* 2013; 131(7):870-9.

[10] Katsimpris, J. M., Petropoulos, I. K., Zoukas, G., Patokos, T., Brinkmann, C. K., Theoulakis, P. E. Central foveal thickness before and after cataract surgery in normal and in diabetic patients without retinopathy. *Klin. Monbl. Augenheilkd.* 2012 Apr.;229(4):331-7.

[11] Jaffe, G. J., Burton, T. C., Kuhn, E., Prescott, A., Hartz, A. Progression of nonproliferative diabetic retinopathy and visual outcome after extracapsular cataract extraction and intraocular lens implantation. *Am. J. Ophthalmol.* 1992 Oct.15;114(4):448-56.

[12] Ostri, C., Lund-Andersen, H., Sander, B., La Cour, M. Phacoemulsification cataract surgery in a large cohort of diabetes patients: visual acuity outcomes and prognostic factors. *J. Cataract Refract. Surg.* 2011 Nov.;37(11):2006-12.

[13] Henricsson, M., Heijl, A., Janzon, L. Diabetic retinopathy before and after cataract surgery. *Br. J. Ophthalmol.* 1996 Sep.;80(9):789-93.

[14] Biro, Z., Balla, Z. Foveal and perifoveal retinal thickness measured by OCT in diabetic patients after phacoemulsification cataract surgery. *Oftalmologia.* 2009;53(2):54-60.

[15] Eriksson, U., Alm, A., Bjarnhall, G., Granstam, E., Matsson, A. W. Macular edema and visual outcome following cataract surgery in patients with diabetic retinopathy and controls. *Graefes Arch. Clin. Exp. Ophthalmol.* 2011 Mar.;249(3):349-59.

[16] Hykin, P. G., Gregson, R. M., Stevens, J. D., Hamilton, P. A. Extracapsular cataract extraction in proliferative diabetic retinopathy. *Ophthalmology*. 1993 Mar.;100(3):394-9.

[17] Meyer, C. H. Current treatment approaches in diabetic macular edema. *Ophthalmologica*. 2007;221(2):118-31.

[18] Patel, J. I., Hykin, P. G., Cree, I. A. Diabetic cataract removal: postoperative progression of maculopathy--growth factor and clinical analysis. *Br. J. Ophthalmol.* 2006 Jun.;90(6):697-701.

[19] Funatsu, H., Yamashita, H., Noma, H., Shimizu, E., Mimura, T., Hori, S. Prediction of macular edema exacerbation after phacoemulsification in patients with nonproliferative diabetic retinopathy. *J. Cataract Refract. Surg.* 2002 Aug.;28(8):1355.

[20] Hartnett, M. E., Tinkham, N., Paynter, L., Geisen, P., Rosenberg, P., Koch, G., et al. Aqueous vascular endothelial growth factor as a predictor of macular thickening following cataract surgery in patients with diabetes mellitus. *Am. J. Ophthalmol.* 2009 Dec.;148(6):895-901 e1.

[21] Campochiaro, P. A., Wykoff, C. C., Shapiro, H., Rubio, R. G., Ehrlich, J. S. Neutralization of Vascular Endothelial Growth Factor Slows Progression of Retinal Nonperfusion in Patients with Diabetic Macular Edema. *Ophthalmology*. 2014 Apr. 23.

[22] *Diabetic Retinopathy Guidelines. December 2012*. The Royal College of Ophthalmologists; 2012 [9th June 2014]; Available from: http://www.rcophth.ac.uk/page.asp?section=451.

[23] Pareja-Rios, A., Serrano-Garcia, M. A., Marrero-Saavedra, M. D., Abraldes-Lopez, V. M., Reyes-Rodriguez, M. A., Cabrera-Lopez, F., et al. [Guidelines of clinical practice of the SERV (Spanish Retina and Vitreous Society): management of ocular complications of diabetes. Diabetic retinopathy and macular oedema]. *Arch. Soc. Esp. Oftalmol.* 2009 Sep.;84(9):429-50.

[24] Jurecka, T., Batkova, Z., Ventruba, J., Synek, S. [Macular edema after cataract surgery in diabetic patients without retinopathy]. *Cesk. Slov. Oftalmol.* 2007 Jul.;63(4):274-84.

[25] *The Effect of Intravitral Injection of Triamcinolone Combined With Cataract Surgery (Phacoemulsification) on Diabetic Macular Edema and Diabetic Retinopathy*. [19th May 2014]; Available from: https://clinicaltrials.gov/ct2/show/NCT00849537?term=diabetes%2C+phacoemulsificationandrank=9.

[26] *Intravitreal Injection Versus Sub-Tenon's Infusion of Triamcinolone Acetonide for Refractory Diabetic Macular Edema During Cataract Surgery*. [19th May 2014]; Available from: https://clinicaltrials.gov/ct2/show/NCT00801450?term=diabetes%2C+phacoemulsificationandrank=8.

[27] *Intraoperative Dexamethasone Implant Improves Outcome of Cataract Surgery With Diabetic Macular Edema*. [19th May 2014]; Available from: https://clinicaltrials.gov/ct2/show/NCT01546402?term=diabetes%2C+phacoemulsificationandrank=3.

[28] Grenga, P., Lupo, S., Domanico, D., Vingolo, E. M. Efficacy of intravitreal triamcinolone acetonide in long standing diabetic macular edema: a microperimetry and optical coherence tomography study. *Retina*. 2008 Oct.;28(9):1270-5.

[29] Cunningham, E. T., Jr., Adamis, A. P., Altaweel, M., Aiello, L. P., Bressler, N. M., D'Amico, D. J., et al. A phase II randomized double-masked trial of pegaptanib, an anti-vascular endothelial growth factor aptamer, for diabetic macular edema. *Ophthalmology*. 2005 Oct.;112(10):1747-57.

[30] Stefanini, F. R., Arevalo, J. F., Maia, M. Bevacizumab for the management of diabetic macular edema. *World J. Diabetes*. 2013 Apr. 15;4(2):19-26.

[31] Malgorzata, W., Diana, D., Agnieszka, B., Zofia, M. Bevacizumab intravitreal injections in the treatment of diabetic macular oedema. *Klin. Oczna*. 2013;115(1):15-9.

[32] Arevalo, J. F., Sanchez, J. G., Lasave, A. F., Wu, L., Maia, M., Bonafonte, S., et al. Intravitreal Bevacizumab (Avastin) for Diabetic Retinopathy: The 2010 GLADAOF Lecture. *J. Ophthalmol*. 2011;2011:584238.

[33] Do, D. V., Nguyen, Q. D., Khwaja, A. A., Channa, R., Sepah, Y. J., Sophie, R., et al. Ranibizumab for edema of the macula in diabetes study: 3-year outcomes and the need for prolonged frequent treatment. *JAMA Ophthalmol*. 2013 Feb.;131(2):139-45.

[34] Mitchell, P., Bandello, F., Schmidt-Erfurth, U., Lang, G. E., Massin, P., Schlingemann, R. O., et al. The RESTORE study: ranibizumab monotherapy or combined with laser versus laser monotherapy for diabetic macular edema. *Ophthalmology*. 2011 Apr.;118(4):615-25.

[35] Moradi, A., Sepah, Y. J., Sadiq, M. A., Nasir, H., Kherani, S., Sophie, R., et al. Vascular endothelial growth factor trap-eye (Aflibercept) for

the management of diabetic macular edema. *World J. Diabetes*. 2013 Dec. 15;4(6):303-9.

[36] Suto, C., Hori, S., Kato, S. Management of type 2 diabetics requiring panretinal photocoagulation and cataract surgery. *J. Cataract Refract. Surg*. 2008 Jun.;34(6):1001-6.

[37] Ram, J., Agarwal, A. K., Gupta, A. Phacoemulsification and intraocular lens implantation after inadvertent intracapsular injection of intravitreal dexamethasone implant. *BMJ Case Rep*. 2012;2012.

[38] Jonas, J. B., Kreissig, I., Degenring, R. Intravitreal triamcinolone acetonide for treatment of intraocular proliferative, exudative, and neovascular diseases. *Prog. Retin. Eye Res*. 2005 Sep.;24(5):587-611.

[39] Kim, S. Y., Yang, J., Lee, Y. C., Park, Y. H. Effect of a single intraoperative sub-Tenon injection of triamcinolone acetonide on the progression of diabetic retinopathy and visual outcomes after cataract surgery. *J. Cataract Refract. Surg*. 2008 May;34(5):823-6.

[40] Habib, M. S., Cannon, P. S., Steel, D. H. The combination of intravitreal triamcinolone and phacoemulsification surgery in patients with diabeticfoveal oedema and cataract. *BMC Ophthalmol*. 2005;5:15.

[41] Ahmadabadi, H. F., Mohammadi, M., Beheshtnejad, H., Mirshahi, A. Effect of intravitreal triamcinolone acetonide injection on central macular thickness in diabetic patients having phacoemulsification. *J. Cataract Refract. Surg*. 2010 Jun.;36(6):917-22.

[42] Beer, P. M., Bakri, S. J., Singh, R. J., Liu, W., Peters, G. B., 3rd, Miller, M. Intraocular concentration and pharmacokinetics of triamcinolone acetonide after a single intravitreal injection. *Ophthalmology*. 2003 Apr.; 110(4):681-6.

[43] Lam, D. S., Chan, C. K., Mohamed, S., Lai, T. Y., Lee, V. Y., Lai, W. W., et al. Phacoemulsification with intravitreal triamcinolone in patients with cataract and coexisting diabetic macular oedema: a 6-month prospective pilot study. *Eye* (Lond.). 2005 Aug.;19(8):885-90.

[44] A randomized trial comparing intravitreal triamcinolone acetonide and focal/grid photocoagulation for diabetic macular edema. *Ophthalmology*. 2008 Sep.;115(9):1447-9, 9 e1-10.

[45] Rauen, P. I., Ribeiro, J. A., Almeida, F. P., Scott, I. U., Messias, A., Jorge, R. Intravitreal injection of ranibizumab during cataract surgery in patients with diabetic macular edema. *Retina*. 2012 Oct.;32(9):1799-803.

[46] Udaondo, P., Garcia-Pous, M., Garcia-Delpech, S., Salom, D., Diaz-Llopis, M. Prophylaxis of macular edema with intravitreal ranibizumab

in patients with diabetic retinopathy after cataract surgery: a pilot study. *J. Ophthalmol.* 2011;2011:159436.

[47] Wahab, S., Ahmed, J. Management of cataract with macular oedema due to diabetes mellitus type-II and hypertension with grid laser prior to surgery and intra-vitreal bevacizumab (Avastin) peroperatively. *J. Pak. Med. Assoc.* 2010 Oct.;60(10):836-9.

[48] Lanzagorta-Aresti, A., Palacios-Pozo, E., Menezo Rozalen, J. L., Navea-Tejerina, A. Prevention of vision loss after cataract surgery in diabetic macular edema with intravitreal bevacizumab: a pilot study. *Retina.* 2009 Apr.;29(4):530-5.

[49] Takamura, Y., Kubo, E., Akagi, Y. Analysis of the effect of intravitreal bevacizumab injection on diabetic macular edema after cataract surgery. *Ophthalmology.* 2009 Jun.;116(6):1151-7.

[50] Chen, C. H., Liu, Y. C., Wu, P. C. The combination of intravitreal bevacizumab and phacoemulsification surgery in patients with cataract and coexisting diabetic macular edema. *J. Ocul. Pharmacol. Ther.* 2009 Feb.;25(1):83-9.

[51] Kern, T. S., Miller, C. M., Du, Y., Zheng, L., Mohr, S., Ball, S. L., et al. Topical administration of nepafenac inhibits diabetes-induced retinal microvascular disease and underlying abnormalities of retinal metabolism and physiology. *Diabetes.* 2007 Feb.;56(2):373-9.

[52] Wolf, E. J., Braunstein, A., Shih, C., Braunstein, R. E. Incidence of visually significant pseudophakic macular edema after uneventful phacoemulsification in patients treated with nepafenac. *J. Cataract Refract. Surg.* 2007 Sep.;33(9):1546-9.

In: Macular Edema
Editor: Earl Davison
ISBN: 978-1-63321-584-9


*Chapter 4*

# MANAGEMENT OF DIABETIC MACULAR EDEMA

***Francisco J. Ascaso, M.D., Ph.D.*** [1,2*]**,**
***Valentín Huerva, M.D., Ph.D.*** [3, 4]
***and Jordi Soldevila, Ph.D.*** [3]
[1]Department of Ophthalmology,
"Lozano Blesa" University Clinic Hospital, Zaragoza, Spain
[2]Aragon Health Sciences Institute, Zaragoza, Spain
[3]Department of Ophthalmology, Universitary Hospital Arnau de Vilanova, Lleida, Spain
[4]IRB-Lleida, Lleida, Spain

## ABSTRACT

Diabetic macular edema (DME) is the main cause of visual impairment in patients with diabetes mellitus (DM). For many years macular laser photocoagulation has been the golf standard therapy for preventing severe visual loss in patients with DME. However, intravitreal pharmacological therapies have changed how DME is managed, improving visual function with a well-documented tolerable safety profile, and providing patients with significant visual acuity gains that are sustainable with repeat injections. Thus, it has been proposed the use of

* Corresponding author´s Email: jascaso@gmail.com.

anti-VEGF or corticosteroids agents as the first line of treatment instead of laser therapy in patients with center-involving DME with moderate visual impairment. Patients who do not yet meet the treatment threshold should be managed with laser therapy according to ETDRS guidelines. On the other hand, although further researches are necessary to establish the best way to care DME patients, and given its multifactorial nature, combination therapy of anti-VEGF drugs with corticosteroids is an evolving field in an effort to alleviate the treatment burden of monthly dosing and to assess the efficacy in those individuals with persistent DME despite repeated anti-VEGF injections.

## INTRODUCTION

Diabetes mellitus (DM) appears to be a global epidemic in the new century that affects over 350 million people worldwide. By 2030, this number is expected to increase to 552 million. [1] This disorder is associated with significant morbidity. Thus, diabetic retinopathy (DR), which is the most common microvascular complication of DM, [2, 3] is present in approximately 30% of diabetic patients, and one in three of DR are at risk of severe vision loss secondary to advanced disease. [4] In fact, DR is the fifth-leading cause of the world's blindness and the more frequent cause of vision loss in working-aged adults. [5-7] There are two groups of DR: proliferative diabetic retinopathy (PDR) and nonproliferative diabetic retinopathy (NPDR). Although PDR leads to a more severe vision loss, the higher prevalence of NPDR results in a larger number of blind people. NPDR is currently classified as mild, moderate, or severe. [8] The last stage is based on the so-called 4:2:1 rule, which consists in at least one of the following findings: diffuse intraretinal hemorrhages in all quadrants, venous beading in at least two quadrants, or the presence of intraretinal microvascular abnormalities (IRMAs) in one or more quadrants. [9]

The most common cause of impairment in visual acuity in NPDR is due to diabetic macular edema (DME), whose prevalence ranges from 3 to 5%, with this percentage increasing with age. [10] DME is defined as an advanced, vision-limiting manifestation of DR in which a breakdown of the blood–retinal barrier, followed by extracellular fluid accumulation may lead to thickening of the retinal tissue in the macular area causing loss of central vision. [11-13] This swelling of the central retina is caused by an abnormal permeability of the perifoveal retinal capillaries, and not explained by an epiretinal membrane (ERM). [14, 15] DME is diagnosed by slit-lamp biomicroscopy and fluorescein angiography. More recently, central macular thickness (CMT) measured by optical coherence tomography (OCT) has become the mainstay used to objectively assess and quantify DME. [9] According to the International Clinical Classification Scale DME is classified in mild, moderate and severe. [16]

During the last 30 years, macular laser photocoagulation has been the gold standard of treatment in patients with clinically significant macular edema (CSME) [17, 18] Nevertheless, there have been important advances in the treatment of DME since intravitreal therapies with steroids or anti–vascular endothelial growth factor (anti-VEGF) are becoming more popular whether used alone or in combination with laser treatments, [19] with visual acuity outcomes surpassing the results obtained with laser alone. [20] Nevertheless, treatment benefits decrease sharply if the therapy is applied too late. [21] The treatment algorithm for selecting diabetic patients, the initiation of corticosteroid or anti-VEGF therapy, and the management of DME using this kind of alternative treatments has not yet been established. This review chapter summarizes major studies and randomized controlled trials (RCTs) examining DME treatment possibilities with the purpose of providing an initial set of evidence-based guidelines for DME treatment.

## Management of Systemic Risk Factors

Duration and control of DM are key components of the primary prevention of DR. Thus, intensive control of blood glucose levels, blood pressure and lipid profile delay and even prevent the onset and progression of DR, and possibly have a major effect on DME. [22-24]

## Laser Photocoagulation for DME

Laser photocoagulation has typically been used to manage DME, but the exact mechanism by which macular laser has an effect remains poorly understood. [25] In 1985, the Early Treatment Diabetic Retinopathy Study (ETDRS) randomized trial found that macular (focal/grid) photocoagulation decreased the risk of moderate to severe loss of visual acuity (VA) from DME by 50% after three years compared with untreated patients. [17] Since then, the use of laser photocoagulation has been the gold standard of treatment for

CSME for two decades. [15] The purpose of focal macular laser photocoagulation is to maintain VA and prevent severe visual loss (≥15 ETDRS letters, or 3 Snellen lines of VA) over the long term. [9] Nevertheless, less than 3% of patients underwent laser therapy experienced visual improvement of 15 letters from baseline, or three lines on the ETDRS scale, and a significant percentage of patients suffer progressive worsening of VA. [26-28] Moreover, long-term use of this therapy has significant risks and adverse effects, such as central and color vision loss, paracentral scotomata, delayed enlargement of laser scars, and occasional secondary choroidal neovascularization (CNV). [29-31]

There are some evidences that very short duration focal macular laser photocoagulation and subthreshold micropulse diode laser therapies are just as efficacious as the modified ETDRS method of laser therapy for DME, but with less adverse effects and a lower risk of inducing CNV; therefore, minimizing scar formation into the foveal region. [20, 32-33] Nevertheless, long-term follow-up is needed to define their precise roles in DME therapy.

## Pharmacological DME Treatment

### Vascular Endothelial Growth Factor (VEGF) Inhibitors

VEGF, considered one of the most powerful mediating agents in the etiology of DME, is upregulated in hypoxic and hyperglycemic conditions and plays an important role in vascular permeability. [9, 15] There is evidence that elevated VEGF intraocular levels are correlated significantly with DME severity. [34] The human VEGF family includes five related molecules: VEGF-A, VEGF-B, VEGF-C, VEGF-D and placental growth factor (PGF). [35-37] VEGF-A (usually known as VEGF) is the best characterized, and is mainly responsible for the angiogenic mechanisms and vasopermeability in humans. [35-36] It is well known that VEGF inhibitors not only reverse visual impairment, stabilizing and preventing future vision loss, but improve visual acuity and restore retinal morphology in patients with DME. [38-47]

Four anti-VEGF drugs, administered by intravitreal injection, are currently used to treat DME: pegaptanib (Macugen®; Eyetech Pharmaceuticals, Palm Beach Gardens, FL, USA), bevacizumab (Avastin®, Genentech, Inc., San Francisco, CA, US), ranibizumab (Lucentis®; Genentech, Inc., San Francisco, CA, US), and aflibercept (Eylea®; Regeneron, Tarrytown, NY). [48-50] Table 1 lists the results of the major studies evaluating anti-VEGF drugs for treating

DME. [48, 51-58] Pegaptanib sodium is a pegylated 28-base RNA aptamer covalently linked to two branched 20 kDa polyethylene glycol moieties (molecular weight of ~50 kDa) that targets potently and specifically the VEGF- 165 isoform, when administered intravitreally every six weeks was found to be more effective than macular laser at two years, with ETDRS letter gains of 6.1 and 1.3, respectively. [49, 59] Bevacizumab, which is a 149 kDa full-length, recombinant, humanized monoclonal antibody that binds all isoforms of VEGF-A, [37, 60] was found to be more efficacious than macular laser for persistent DME at two years, with ETDRS letter gains of 8.5 and −0.5, respectively. [48] Neither pegaptanib nor bevacizumab is approved by the Food and Drug Administration (FDA) to treat DME. [9] Pegaptanib (Macugen® package insert) is approved for the treatment of neovascular AMD by the US FDA. [25] Bevacizumab is neither designed nor manufactured for intraocular use; nevertheless, it is used off-label, by intravitreal injection, for treating retinal vascular diseases, such as neovascular age-related macular degeneration (AMD), retinal vein occlusion (RVO), and DME. [37] In August 2012, ranibizumab (Lucentis®, Genentech, Inc., South San Francisco, CA, USA), a 48 kDa recombinant humanized monoclonal anti-VEGF antigen fragment that binds all VEGF-A isoforms, [60] was approved by the FDA to treat DME at the 0.3mg dose, administered monthly by intravitreal injection. [9] It is specifically designed and manufactured for using into the eye (Lucentis® package insert), and is the only anti-VEGF agent approved for treating DME. [60, 61] The ranibizumab molecule also lacks a Fc region, which allows for shorter systemic circulation and faster clearance. [60] Ranibizumab therapy resulted in almost 40% of eyes with visually significant DME gaining ≥15 ETDRS letters or more of vision compared to only 18% of control eyes. The mean VA gain with monthly intravitreal ranibizumab injections was 10.9 and 12 ETDRS letters in the 0.3mg and 0.5mg groups, respectively, compared to a 2.3 letter gain in the control group. Results were sustained for 24 months with continued therapy. [52] The most recent VEGF inhibitor which has been introduced is aflibercept (Eylea®, Regeneron Pharmaceuticals, Inc., Tarrytown, NY, USA), previously known as the VEGF-Trap-Eye. [9] It is a 115 kDa recombinant fusion protein consisting of portions of the human VEGFR-1 and VEGFR-2 fused to the Fc domain of human immunoglobulin G1 domain (Eylea package insert). [62] Aflibercept is currently approved in the US and Europe for the treatment of neovascular AMD and CRVO-associated ME. It binds all isoforms of VEGF-A, VEGF-B, and PGF, is delivered by intravitreal injection and is currently under study for treating DME. [36, 62] The results at first year demonstrated that over 40% of eyes with visually significant DME gained at least 15 ETDRS letters of vision compared to 11.4% in the macular laser control group. [57]

## Table 1. Results of the major studies evaluating anti-VEGF drugs for treating DME

| Treatment | Randomized Controlled Trial (n eyes) | Study Design and Duration | Treatment Arms (n) | Mean ± SD (Where Available) VA at Baseline | Mean ± SD (Where Available) ETDRS Letter Change From Baseline | Proportion of Patients With BCVA Change (%): ≥10 Letters Gained | ≥10 Letters Lost | ≥15 Letters Gained | ≥15 Letters Lost | Licensed Indication for Ophthalmic Use |
|---|---|---|---|---|---|---|---|---|---|---|
| **Anti-VEGF agents** | | | | | | | | | | |
| RBZ | RESOLVE (151)[56] | Phase II, 12 months | **Study treatment**: | | | | | | | Yes |
| | | | 0.3/0.6 mg RBZ (51)<br>0.5/1.0 mg RBZ (51) | 60.2 ± 9.9 | RBZ pooled: 7.8 ± 7.7 | RBZ pooled: 60.8 | RBZ pooled: 4.9 | RBZ pooled: 32.4 | RBZ pooled: 2.9 | |
| | | | **Comparator:** | | | | | | | |
| | | | Sham (49) | 61.1 ± 9.0 | Sham: -0.1 ± 9.8 | Sham: 8.4 | Sham: 24.5 | Sham: 10.2 | Sham: 20.4 | |
| | READ-2 (126)[55] | Phase II, 24 months | **Study treatment**: | | | | | | | |
| | | | 0.5 mg RBZ (33) | 24.85 | 0.5 mg RBZ: 7.7 | 0.5 mg RBZ: 43 | N/A | 0.5 mg RBZ: 25 | N/A | |
| | | | **Comparator:** | | | | | | | |
| | | | Laser (34) | 23.83 | Laser: 5.1 | Laser: 23% | | Laser: 9 | | |
| | | | 0.5 mg RBZ + laser (34) | 24.84 | 0.5 mg RBZ + laser: 6.8 | 0.5 mg RBZ + laser: 38 | | 0.5 mg + laser: 7 | | |
| | READ-2 (126)[91] | Phase II, 36 months | **Study treatment**: | | | | | | | |
| | | | 0.5 mg RBZ (28) | N/A | 0.5 mg RBZ: 10.3 | 0.5 mg RBZ: 46 | N/A | 0.5 mg RBZ: 32 | N/A | |
| | | | **Comparator:** | | | | | | | |
| | | | Laser (22) | | Laser: 1.4 | Laser: 23% | | Laser: 9 | | |
| | | | 0.5 mg RBZ + laser (24) | | 0.5 mg RBZ + laser: 8.9 | 0.5 mg RBZ + laser: 38 | | 0.5 mg RBZ + laser: 21 | | |
| | RESTORE (345)[53] | Phase III, 12 months | **Study treatment**: | | | | | | | |
| | | | 0.5 mg RBZ (116)<br>0.5 mg RBZ + laser (118) | 64.8 ± 10.11<br>63.4 ± 9.99 | 0.5 mg RBZ: 6.1 ± 6.43<br>0.5 mg RBZ + laser: 5.9 ± 7.92 | 0.5 mg RBZ: 37.4<br>0.5 mg RBZ + laser: 43.2 | 0.5 mg RBZ: 3.5<br>0.5 mg RBZ + laser: 4.2 | 0.5 mg RBZ: 22.6<br>0.5 mg RBZ + laser: 27.9 | 0.5 mg RBZ: 0.9<br>0.5 mg RBZ + laser: 3.4 | |
| | | | **Comparator:** | | | | | | | |
| | | | Laser (111) | 62.4 ± 11.11 | Laser: 0.8 ± 8.56 | Laser: 15.5 | Laser: 12.7 | Laser: 8.2 | Laser: 8.2 | |
| | DRCR.net Protocol I (854 eyes)[44] | Phase III, 60 months | **Study treatment:**[a] | | **At 12 months**: | | | | | |
| | | | 0.5 mg RBZ + prompt laser (187 eyes) | 63 ± 12 | 0.5 mg RBZ + prompt laser: +9 ± 11 | 0.5 mg RBZ + prompt laser: 30 | 0.5 mg RBZ + prompt laser: 50 | 0.5 mg RBZ + prompt laser: 4 | 0.5 mg RBZ + prompt laser: 2% | |
| | | | 0.5 mg RBZ + deferred laser (188 eyes) | | 0.5 mg RBZ + deferred laser: +9 ± 12 | 0.5 mg RBZ + deferred laser: 28 | 0.5 mg RBZ + deferred laser: 47 | 0.5 mg RBZ + deferred laser: 3 | 0.5 mg RBZ + deferred laser: 2 | |
| | | | **Comparator:** | | | | | | | |
| | | | 4 mg TA + prompt | | 4 mg TA + prompt | 4 mg TA + prompt | 4 mg TA + prompt | 4 mg TA + prompt | 4 mg TA + prompt | |

| Treatment | Randomized Controlled Trial (n) | Study Design and Duration | Treatment Arms (n) | Mean ± SD (Where Available) VA at Baseline | Mean ± SD (Where Available) ETDRS Letter Change From Baseline | Proportion of Patients With BCVA Change (%) ≥10 Letters Gained | ≥10 Letters Lost | ≥15 Letters Gained | ≥15 Letters Lost | Licensed Indication for Ophthalmic Use |
|---|---|---|---|---|---|---|---|---|---|---|
| | | | Sham + prompt laser (293 eyes) | | Sham injection + prompt laser: 3 ± 13 | Sham injection + prompt laser: 15 | Sham injection + prompt laser: 28 | Sham injection + prompt laser: 13 | Sham injection + prompt laser: 8 | |
| | DRCR.net Protocol I (642 eyes)[45] | Phase III, 60 months | **Study treatment:** | | **At 24 months:** | | | | | |
| | | | 0.5 mg RBZ + prompt laser (136 eyes) | 63 ± 13 | 0.5 mg RBZ + prompt laser: +7 ± 13 | 0.5 mg RBZ + prompt laser: 44 | 0.5 mg RBZ + prompt laser: 7 | 0.5 mg RBZ + prompt laser: 29 | 0.5 mg RBZ + prompt laser: 4 | |
| | | | 0.5 mg RBZ + deferred laser (139 eyes) | 63 ± 11 | 0.5 mg RBZ + deferred laser: 9 ± 14 | 0.5 mg RBZ + deferred laser: 49 | 0.5 mg RBZ + deferred laser: 3 | 0.5 mg RBZ + deferred laser: 28 | 0.5 mg RBZ + deferred laser: 2 | |
| | | | **Comparator:** | | | | | | | |
| | | | 4 mg TA + prompt laser (142 eyes) | 64 ± 11 | 4 mg TA + prompt laser: 2 ± 19 | 4 mg TA + prompt laser: 41 | 4 mg TA + prompt laser: 19 | 4 mg TA + prompt laser: 22 | 4 mg TA + prompt laser: 13 | |
| | | | Sham + prompt laser (211 eyes) | 63 ± 12 | Sham + prompt laser: 3 ± 15 | Sham + prompt laser: 36 | Sham + prompt laser: 13 | Sham + prompt laser: 18 | Sham + prompt laser: 10 | |
| | DRCR.net Protocol I (361 eyes)[46] | Phase III, 60 months | **Study treatment:** | | **At 36 months:** | **At 36 months:** | **At 36 months:** | **At 36 months:** | **At 36 months:** | |
| | | | 0.5 mg RBZ + prompt laser (144 eyes) | N/A | 0.5 mg RBZ + prompt laser: 7 ± 12 | 0.5 mg RBZ + prompt laser: 41 | 0.5 mg RBZ + prompt laser: 11 | 0.5 mg RBZ + prompt laser: 26 | 0.5 mg RBZ + prompt laser: 6 | |
| | | | 0.5 mg RBZ + deferred laser (147 eyes) | | 0.5 mg RBZ + deferred laser: 10 ± 11 | 0.5 mg RBZ + deferred: 56 | 0.5 mg RBZ + deferred laser: 5 | 0.5 mg RBZ + deferred laser: 32 | 0.5 mg RBZ + deferred laser: 3 | |
| | RISE (377)[90] | Phase III, 24 months | **Study treatment:** | | | | | | | |
| | | | 0.3 mg RBZ (125) | 54.7 ± 12.6 | 0.3 mg RBZ: 12.5 ± 14.1 | 0.3 mg RBZ: 62.7 | 0.3 mg RBZ: 3.2 | 0.3 mg RBZ: 44.8 | 0.3 mg RBZ: 2.4 | |
| | | | 0.5 mg RBZ (125) | 56.9 ± 11.6 | 0.5 mg RBZ: 11.9 ± 12.1 | 0.5 mg RBZ: 62.4 | 0.5 mg RBZ: 4.0 | 0.5 mg RBZ: 39.2 | 0.5 mg RBZ: 2.4 | |
| | | | **Comparator:** | | | | | | | |
| | | | Sham (127) | 57.2 ± 11.1 | Sham: 2.6 ± 13.9 | Sham: 29.9 | Sham: 16.6 | Sham: 18.1 | Sham: 10.3 | |
| | RIDE (382)[90] | Phase III, 24 months | **Study treatment:** | | | | | | | |
| | | | 0.3 mg RBZ (125) | 57.5 ± 11.6 | 0.3 mg RBZ: 10.9 ± 10.4 | 0.3 mg RBZ: 59.2 | 0.3 mg RBZ: 3.2 | 0.3 mg RBZ: 33.6 | 0.3 mg RBZ: 1.6 | |
| | | | 0.5 mg RBZ (127) | 56.9 ± 11.8 | 0.5 mg RBZ: 12.0 ± 14.9 | 0.5 mg RBZ: 64.5 | 0.5 mg RBZ: 4.0 | 0.5 mg RBZ: 45.7 | 0.5 mg RBZ: 4.0 | |
| | | | **Comparator:** | | | | | | | |
| | | | Sham (130) | 57.3 ± 11.2 | Sham: 2.3 ± 14.2 | Sham: 25.4 | Sham: 13.8 | Sham: 12.3 | Sham: 8.4 | |

## Table 1. (Continued)

| Treatment | Randomized Controlled Trial (n) | Study Design and Duration | Treatment Arms (n) | Mean ± SD (Where Available) VA at Baseline | Mean ± SD (Where Available) ETDRS Letter Change From Baseline | Proportion of Patients With BCVA Change (%) | | | | Licensed Indication for Ophthalmic Use |
|---|---|---|---|---|---|---|---|---|---|---|
| | | | | | | ≥10 Letters Gained | ≥10 Letters Lost | ≥15 Letters Gained | ≥15 Letters Lost | |
| Bevacizumab | BOLT (80)[48] | Phase II, 24 months | **Study treatment:** | | **At 12 months:** | | | | | No |
| | | | ivB (42) | 55.7± 9.7 | ivB: 8 (IQR 1-10) | ivB: 31.0 | N/A | ivB: 11.9 | N/A | |
| | | | **Comparator:** | | | | | | | |
| | | | Laser (38) | 54.6 ± 8.6 | Laser: -0.5 (IQR -15-5) | Laser: 7.9 | | Laser: 5.3 | | |
| | | | **Study treatment:** | | **At 24 months:** | | | | | |
| | | | ivB (37) | 55.8 ± 9.7 | 1.25 mg in 0.05 ml ivB: 8.6 ± 9.1 | ivB: 49 | N/A | ivB: 32 | N/A | |
| | | | **Comparator:** | | | | | | | |
| | | | Laser (28) | 5.4 ± 7.9 | Laser: -0.5 ± 10.6 | Laser: 7 | | Laser: 4 | | |
| | Soheilian et al, 2012 (150 eyes)[95] | Phase III, 24 months | **Study treatment:** | (logMAR) | | | | | | |
| | | | ivB (50) | 0.71 ± 0.28 | ivB: -0.10 ± 0.37 | N/A | N/A | ivB: 41.0 | N/A | |
| | | | ivB/TA (50) | 0.73 ± 0.28 | ivB/TA: -0.09 ± 0.33 | | | ivB/TA: 36.1 | | |
| | | | **Comparator:** | | | | | | | |
| | | | Laser (50) | 0.55 ± 0.26 | Laser: 0.03 ± 0.33 | | | Laser: 23.7 | | |
| Aflibercept | DA VINCI (221)[92] | Phase II, 12 months | **Study treatment:** | | **At 52 weeks:** | **At 52 weeks:** | | **At 52 weeks:** | | Yes |
| | | | 0.5 mg q4 (44) | 59.3 ± 11.2 | 0.5 mg q4: 11.0 | 0.5 mg q4: 57 | N/A | 0.5 mg q4: 40.9 | N/A | |
| | | | 2 mg q4 (44) | 59.9 ± 10.1 | 2 mg q4: 13.0 | 2 mg q4: 71 | | 2 mg q4: 45.5 | | |
| | | | 2 mg q8 (42) | 58.8 ± 12.2 | 2 mg q8: 9.7 | 2 mg q8: 45 | | 2 mg q8: 23.8 | | |
| | | | 2 mg PRN (45) | 59.6 ± 11.1 | 2 mg PRN: 12.0 | 2 mg PRN: 62 | | 2 mg PRN: 42.2 | | |
| | | | **Comparator:** | | | | | | | |
| | | | Laser (44) | 57.6 ± 12.5 | Laser: -1.3 | Laser: 30 | | Laser: 11.4% | | |
| Pegaptanib | Sultan et al, 2011 (207)[96] | Phase II/III, 2 years | **Study treatment:** | | | | | | | Yes |
| | | | 0.3 mg pegaptanib (107) | 57.0 ± 8.9 | 0.3 mg pegaptanib: 6.1 | 0.3 mg pegaptanib: 38.3 | 0.3 mg pegaptanib: 3.0-3.8 | 0.3 mg pegaptanib: 23.4 | N/A | |
| | | | **Comparator:** | | | | | | | |
| | | | Sham (100) | 57.5 ± 8.1 | Sham: 1.3 | Sham: 30.0 | Sham: 6.3-9.0% | Sham: 15.0 | | |

# Table 2. Outcomes of the major studies evaluating corticosteroids for the management of DME

| Treatment | Randomized Controlled Trial (n eyes) | Study Design and Duration | Treatment Arms (n) | Mean ± SD (Where Available) VA at Baseline | Mean ± SD (Where Available) ETDRS Letter Change From Baseline | Proportion of Patients With BCVA Change (%) | | | | Licensed Indication for Ophthalmic Use |
|---|---|---|---|---|---|---|---|---|---|---|
| | | | | | | ≥10 Letters Gained | ≥10 Letters Lost | ≥15 Letters Gained | ≥15 Letters Lost | |
| **Intravitreal corticosteroids** | | | | | | | | | | |
| Triamcinolone acetonide (TA) | Gillies et al, 2011 (84 eyes)[35] | Phase II/III, 24 months | **Study treatment:** | | | | | | | |
| | | | 4 mg TA + laser (42) | 55.2 ± (12.5) | 4 mg TA + laser: 0.76 | 4 mg TA + laser: 36% | 4 mg TA + laser: 33% | N/A | N/A | |
| | | | **Comparator:** | | | | | | | |
| | | | Laser (42) | 55.5 ± (11.3) | Laser: -1.46 | Laser: 17% | Laser: 24% | | | |
| | Gillies et al, 2006 (69 eyes)[66] | Phase II, 60 months | **Study treatment:** | | **At 24 months:** | **At 24 months:** | **At 24 months:** | **At 24 months:** | **At 24 months:** | Yes |
| | | | 4 mg TA (34 eyes) | 60.5 ± 11.9 | 4 mg TA: 3.1 | 4 mg TA: 21 | 4 mg TA: 9% | 4 mg TA: 12 | 4 mg TA: 3 | |
| | | | **Comparator:** | | | | | | | |
| | | | Placebo (35 eyes) | 61.3 ± 13.2 | Placebo: -2.9 | Placebo: 12 | Placebo: 25 | Placebo: 3 | Placebo: 11 | |
| | | | **Study treatment:** | | **At 60 months:** | **At 60 months:** | **At 60 months:** | | | |
| | | | 4 mg TA (33 eyes) | 59.0 ± 11.7 | 4 mg TA: -1.8 | 4 mg TA: 27% | 4 mg TA: 18 | N/A | N/A | |
| | | | **Comparator:** | | | | | | | |
| | | | Placebo (34 eyes) | 59.5 ± 14.0 | Placebo: -2.7 | Placebo: 18 | Placebo: 24 | | | |
| | DRCR.net (693)[24] | Phase III, 24 months | **Study treatment:** | | | | | | | |
| | | | 1 mg TA (256) | Pooled: 59±11 | 1 mg TA: -2±18 | 1 mg TA: 25 | 1 mg TA: 26 | 1 mg TA: 14 | 1 mg TA: 20 | |
| | | | 4 mg TA (254) | | 4 mg TA: -3±22 | 4 mg TA: 28 | 4 mg TA: 28 | 4 mg TA: 17 | 4 mg TA: 20 | |
| | | | **Comparator:** | | | | | | | |
| | | | Laser (330) | | Laser: 1 ± 17 | Laser: 31 | Laser: 19 | Laser: 18 | Laser: 14 | |
| Fluocinolone acetonide | FAME (956)[26,27] | Phase III, 36 months | **Study treatment:** | | **At 24 months:** | | | **At 24 months:** | | Yes |
| | | | 0.2 μg/day (185) | 53.3 ± 12.69 | 0.2 μg/day = +4.4 | N/A | N/A | 0.2 μg/day = 26.1 | N/A | |
| | | | 0.5 μg/day (375) | 52.9 ± 12.21 | 0.5 μg/day = +5.4 | | | 0.5 μg/day = 26.7 | | |
| | | | **Comparator:** | | | | | | | |
| | | | Sham injection (393) | 54.7 ± 11.27 | Sham = +1.7 | | | Sham = 13% | | |
| | | | | | **At 36 months:** | | | **At 36 months:** | | |
| | | | | | 0.2 μg/day = +7.6 | N/A | N/A | 0.2 μg/day = 28.7 | N/A | |
| | | | | | 0.5 μg/day = +6.2 | | | 0.5 μg/day = 27.8 | | |
| | | | | | Sham = +1.8 | | | Sham = 18.9 | | |

**Table 2. (Continued)**

0.5 mg q4 = 0.5 mg VEGF Trap-Eye every 4 weeks; 2 mg q4 = 2 mg VEGF Trap-Eye every 4 weeks; 2 mg q8 = 2 mg VEGF Trap-Eye for 3 initial monthly doses and then every 8 weeks; 2 mg PRN =2 mg VEGF Trap-Eye for 3 initial monthly doses and then on an as-needed basis; BCVA = best-corrected visual acuity; BOLT = Bevacizumab or Laser Therapy; DA VINCI = DME and VEGF Trap-Eye; DRCR.net = Diabetic Retinopathy Clinical Research Network; ETDRS = Early Treatment Diabetic Retinopathy Study; FAME = Fluocinolone Acetonide in Diabetic Macular Edema; IQR = inter- quartile range; ivB = intravitreal bevacizumab; LogMAR = logarithm of the minimal angle of resolution; PRN = pro re nata; N/A = not available; READ-2 = Two-year Outcomes of the Ranibizumab for Edema of the macula in Diabetes; RESOLVE = Safety and Efficacy of Ranibizumab in Diabetic Macular Edema; RESTORE = A 12 Month Core Study to Assess the Efficacy and Safety of Ranibi- zumab Intravitreal Injections; RIDE/RISE = A Study of Ranibizumab Injection in subjects with CSDME with Center Involvement Secondary to Diabetes Mellitus; RBZ = ranibizumab; SD = standard deviation; SOC = standard of care; TA = triamcinolone acetonide; VA = visual acuity; VEGF = vascular endothelial growth factor.

[a] Includes only eyes with VA measurements at baseline and 2-year visit.

## Intravitreal Corticosteroids

Corticosteroids were the first pharmacologic intravitreal therapy to be used for DME. Although their exact mechanism of action is not completely understood, corticosteroids reduce retinal vascular permeability, decreasing the production of arachidonic acid derivatives such as prostaglandins, as well as inhibiting ICAM-1, TNF-$\alpha$, and VEGF and VEGF gene expression. [20, 22, 24, 37]

Triamcinolone acetonide (TA) has been the most widely used and studied corticosteroid in the DME management. [24, 63-67] Intravitreal injection of TA (off label) reduces DME and improves VA; [37] nevertheless, in RCTs, this drug did not showed better results than those with laser photocoagulation in patients with DME. [24, 44]

Sustained delivery systems releasing either fluocinolone or dexamethasone have also been evaluated. There are three commercially available slow-release corticosteroid implants: Retisert®, Iluvien®, and Ozurdex®. Two of the available devices release fluocinolone acetonide (FA), whose low solubility makes it suitable for slow-release without the need for a polymer system. Retisert® (Bausch & Lomb, Rochester, New York, USA) is a sterile, a time-released nonbioerodible surgically implantable reservoir of FA, implanted surgically through a scleral opening in the pars plana. [9] It is licensed by the US FDA, but not by the European Medicines Agency (EMA) for treating chronic noninfectious posterior uveitis. [68] It contains 0.59 mg FA and was designed to release approximately 0.5 mg/day for 1000 days. [69] Iluvien® (Alimera Sciences, Alpharetta, GA, USA) is an injectable intravitreal insert, a nonbioerodible cylindrical polymide tube, delivered using a 25G injector system and designed to release FA gradually for up to three years. [70-72] Iluvien® is available in the UK and France for using in chronic and refractory DME; nevertheless, it has not been approved by the US FDA for this indication. [70] It has been evaluated for the treatment of DME at two doses: 0.2 and 0.5 mg/day. [73] Thus, in a 36-month, sham-controlled double-masked, phase III trial, the efficacy and safety profile of FA was compared with that of sham injection in patients with persistent or recurrent DME. [71, 72] FA showed no benefit in preventing vision loss compared with non-treatment, as similar proportions of patients progressed to blindness (BCVA 20/200 or worse). In another phase II/III study evaluating the efficacy and safety of FA 0.59 mg inserts against standard therapies (i.e., observation or laser treatment), there was no significant difference in the percentage of eyes gaining >15 letters between patients in both arms after three years following implant. [74] The dexamethasone (DEX) drug delivery system commercialized as Ozurdex® (Allergan, Irvine, California, USA) consists of dexamethasone bound with a biodegradable copolymer of lactic and glycolic acids. [67] Injected through the pars plana using a 22G injection system, it is placed into the vitreous cavity and releases 700 mg of dexamethasone gradually for up to six months as the polymer degrades, so therapy can be repeated as needed. [75] Ozurdex is approved by the US FDA and EMA for the treatment of macular edema following branch or central RVO and also for treating noninfectious posterior segment uveitis (Ozurdex® package insert). In the phase II PLACID trial, patients with diffuse DME demonstrated similar visual gains (≥10 letters; two lines on the ETDRS chart) from baseline at month 12 whether treated with the DEX implant plus laser or sham implant plus laser. [75] Nevertheless, increased intraocular pressure (IOP) and cataract-related adverse effects were reported more frequently in the DEX plus laser therapy group compared with sham group. [25]

None of the corticosteroids above mentioned are currently FDA approved to treat DME. [9] Table 2 lists the outcomes of the major studies evaluating corticosteroids for the management of DME. [27, 66, 74, 76-78] The increased incidence of premature cataract formation and IOP increments with intravitreal corticosteroids compared to with sham and laser procedures raises important aspects in clinical practice. [24, 26-28, 66, 79, 80] Although small, the risk for surgical treatments, such as phacoemulsification, laser trabeculoplasty, and glaucoma surgery, increases therapy-related morbidity. [15]

## Combination Therapy for DME Management

Intravitreal pharmacological agents have replaced macular laser therapy as the gold standard in the DME treatment. However, as invasive procedures, they imply numerous physician visits and potential complications. Although further researches are necessary to assess how best to manage DME patients, and given its multifactorial nature, combination treatment of anti-VEGF drugs with corticosteroids is an evolving field in an attempt to relieve the therapy burden of monthly dosing and to evaluate the efficacy in those individuals with persistent DME despite repeated anti-VEGF therapy. [9]

This has inspired studies to estimate if combination regimes with both intravitreal injections and laser can be more effective than either treatment alone or if combination treatment allows for fewer therapies while maintaining VA improvements. According to the Diabetic Retinopathy Clinical Research

Network (DRCR), at the end of the 2-year study, ranibizumab + delayed focal macular laser was the superior treatment algorithm for patients with visually significant DME. In the ranibizumab + delayed laser group 28% of eyes gained ≥15ETDRS (mean gain = 9 letters); in the ranibizumab + prompt laser group 29% of eyes gained ≥15 ETDRS letters (mean gain = 8 letters); a median of only two and three ranibizumab injections were needed the second year for the delayed versus prompt groups, respectively. In the laser only group, 18% of eyes gained ≥15 ETDRS letters with a mean VA improvement of three letters. In the TA + laser group, 22% of eyes gained ≥15 ETDRS letters, with a mean VA gain of 2 letters. [19] A 2-year retrospective study evaluating bevacizumab versus bevacizumab + macular laser versus macular laser alone for patients with DME found that the bevacizumab only group did better than the other groups with gains of 11.8 ETDRS letters compared to 8.2 and 4.8 ETDRS letter gains, respectively. There was no statistically significant difference between the bevacizumab and bevacizumab + macular laser group, but both these groups were statistically superior to the macular laser only group. [51] The main limitation of this study is its retrospective nature. Furthermore, the number of intravitreal injections in the bevacizumab groups was not indicated.

## SURGICAL TREATMENT OF DME

The role of pars plana posterior vitrectomy (PPV) for the treatment of refractory DME is less clear compared with other therapies. Several RCTs have described contradictory results on PPV with and without the removal of the internal limiting membrane in eyes with DME refractory to standard laser therapy. [81-84] Although PPV effectively decreased retinal thickness, visual results were less consistent, with vision improvement in some eyes and worsening of VA in others. The evidence for combining PPV with intravitreal corticosteroids, intravitreal anti-VEGF agents, and/or laser photocoagulation to treat refractory DME is limited to small, nonrandomized, uncontrolled case series. [85-87] Solid proofs from large, well-designed RCTs with long-term follow-up are necessary to confirm a role for this management approach in DME.

# TREATMENT GUIDELINES OF DME

According to several metaanalyses, the use of anti-VEGF agents is an alternative or adjunctive therapy to laser. [88, 89] Thus, the treatment with VEGF inhibitors agents should be considered in center-involving DME and VA ≤ 20/30, as this was the inclusion criteria in the pivotal RCTs of anti-VEGF treatments. [43-47, 56, 90-92]

For patients with DME without center involvement or for center-involving DME with VA ≥ 20/30, focal laser photocoagulation using ETDRS guidelines should still be considered. In fact, there is currently no evidence to support the use of VEGF inhibitors in eyes with VA ≥20/30. Regarding treatment initiation and follow-up regimen, it is recommended a "loading dose" with monthly anti-VEGF injections given for at least three consecutive months followed by monthly assessment visits. [43-47, 93] The rationale for continuing anti-VEGF treatment is that if VA is still improving, or it has decreased due to DME, then injection should be repeated. If VA remained unchanged for at least two consecutive visits, then injections could be interrupted and monthly follow-up continued. The presence on OCT of intraretinal or subretinal fluid, could also guide either the continuation or discontinuation of injections. [93]

When DME is associated with cataract, efforts should be made to resolve the DME before phacoemulsification surgery. [94] The DRCR.net cautions against the long-term use of IVTA owing to increased risk of glaucoma and progression of cataract. [24, 44, 45] Nevertheless, pseudophakic eyes may benefit from combined intravitreal corticosteroids (especially the DEX implant) and laser photocoagulation therapy, although similar results were achieved with ranibizumab plus laser. [44, 46]

# CONCLUSION

DME is the main cause of visual impairment in patients with DM. For many years macular laser photocoagulation has been the primary therapy for preventing severe visual loss in patients with DME. However, intravitreal pharmacological therapies have changed how DME is managed, improving visual function with a well-documented tolerable safety profile, and providing patients with significant VA gains that are sustainable with repeat injections. Thus, it has been proposed the use of anti-VEGF or corticosteroids agents as the first line of treatment instead of laser therapy in patients with center-involving DME with moderate visual impairment. Patients who do not yet meet the treatment threshold should be managed with laser therapy according to ETDRS guidelines. On the other hand, although further researches are necessary to establish the best way to care DME patients, and given its multifactorial nature, combination therapy of anti-VEGF drugs with corticosteroids is an evolving field in an effort to alleviate the treatment burden of monthly dosing and to assess the efficacy in those individuals with persistent DME despite repeated anti-VEGF injections. Finally, macular laser treatment still has a role in DME management, particularly focal DME.

## REFERENCES


[1] International Diabetes Federation. IDF Diabetes Atlas 2011, 5th edition. Available at: http://www.idf.org/diabetesatlas (accessed 11 October 2012).

[2] Fong D, Aiello L, Ferris F, Klein R. Diabetic retinopathy. *Diabetes Care* 2004; 27: 2540-2553.

[3] American Diabetes Association. Standards of medical care in diabetes – 2012. *Diabetes Care* 2012; 35(Suppl. 1): S11–S63.

[4] Sobngwi E, Mauvais-Jarvis F, Vexiau P, Mbanya JC, Gautier JF. Diabetes in Africans. Part 1: epidemiology and clinical specificities. *Diabetes Metab* 2001; 27:628–634.

[5] Moss SE, Klein R, Klein BE. The 14-year incidence of visual loss in a diabetic population. *Ophthalmology* 1998; 105:998-1003.

[6] Cheung N, Mitchell P, Wong TY. Diabetic retinopathy. *Lancet* 2010; 376(9735):124–136.

[7] Centers for Disease Control and Prevention, National Diabetes Fact Sheet: National Estimates and General Information on Diabetes and pre Diabetes in the United States, 2011, Department of Health and Human Services, Centers for Disease Control and Prevention, Atlanta, Ga, USA, 2011.

[8] Jain A, Sarraf D, Fong D. Preventing diabetic retinopathy through control of systemic factors. *Current Opinion in Ophthalmology* 2003; 14:389-394.

[9] Jain A, Varshney N, Smith C. The Evolving Treatment Options for Diabetic Macular Edema. *Int J Inflam* 2013;2013:689276.

[10] Ding J, Wong TY. Current epidemiology of diabetic retinopathy and diabetic macular edema. *Current Diabetes Reports* 2012; 12:346-354.

[11] Frank R. Diabetic retinopathy. *NEJM* 2004; 350:48-58.

[12] Johnson M. Etiology and treatment of macular edema. *Am J Ophthalmol* 2009; 147:11-21.

[13] Miller J, Le Couter J, Strauss E, Ferrara N. Vascular endothelial growth factor A in intraocular vascular disease. *Ophthalmology* 2012; 120:106-114.

[14] Scholl S, Augustin A, Loewenstein A, Rizzo S, Kupperman B. General pathophysiology of macular edema. *Eur J Ophthalmol* 2011;21 Suppl 6:S10-9.

[15] Mitchell P, Wong TY; Diabetic Macular Edema Treatment Guideline Working Group. Management paradigms for diabetic macular edema. *Am J Ophthalmol* 2014;157:505-513.e8.

[16] Wilkinson CP, Ferris FL III, Klein RE, et al; for the Global Diabetic Retinopathy Project Group. Proposed international clinical diabetic retinopathy and diabetic macular edema disease severity scales. *Ophthalmology* 2003;110:1677-1682.

[17] Early Treatment Diabetic Retinopathy Study Research Group. Photocoagulation for diabetic macular edema. ETDRS report number 1. *Arch Ophthalmol* 1985;103:1796-1806.

[18] Aiello LM. Perspectives on diabetic retinopathy. *Am J Ophthalmol* 2003; 136:122-135.

[19] Elman MJ, Bressler NM, Qin H, et al; Diabetic Retinopathy Clinical Research Network. Expanded 2-year follow-up of ranibizumab plus prompt or deferred laser or triamcinolone plus prompt laser for diabetic macular edema. *Ophthalmology* 2011;118:609-614.

[20] Witkin AJ, Brown GC. Update on nonsurgical therapy for diabetic macular edema. *Curr Opin Ophthalmol* 2011;22:185-189.

[21] Stefansson E, Bek T, Porta M, Larsen N, Kristinsson JK, Agardh E. Screening and prevention of diabetic blindness. *Acta Ophthalmol Scand* 2000;78:374-385.

[22] Blumenkranz MS. Optimal current and future treatments for diabetic macular oedema. *Eye* 2010; 24:428-434.

[23] The Diabetes Control and Complications Trial/Epidemiology of Diabetes Interventions and Complications Research Group. Retinopathy and nephropathy in patients with type 1 diabetes four years after a trial of intensive therapy. *NEJM* 2000; 342:381-389.

[24] Diabetic Retinopathy Clinical Research Network. A randomized trial comparing intravitreal triamcinolone acetonide and focal/ grid photocoagulation for diabetic macular edema. *Ophthalmology* 2008; 115:1447-1459.

[25] Boyer DS, Hopkins JJ, Sorof J, Ehrlich JS. Anti-vascular endothelial growth factor therapy for diabetic macular edema. *Ther Adv Endocrinol Metab* 2013;4:151-169.

[26] Campochiaro PA, Brown DM, Pearson A, et al. Long-term benefit of sustained-delivery fluocinolone acetonide vitreous inserts for diabetic macular edema. *Ophthalmology* 2011;118:626-635.e2.

[27] Campochiaro PA, Brown DM, Pearson A, et al; for the FAME Study Group. Sustained delivery fluocinolone acetonide vitreous inserts provide benefit for at least 3 years in patients with diabetic macular edema. *Ophthalmology* 2012; 119:2125-2132.

[28] Pearson PA, Comstock TL, Ip M, et al. Fluocinolone acetonide intravitreal implant for diabetic macular edema: a 3- year multicenter, randomized, controlled clinical trial. *Ophthalmology* 2011;118:1580-1587.

[29] Luttrull JK, Dorin G. Subthreshold diode micropulse laser photocoagulation (SDM) as invisible retinal phototherapy for diabetic macular edema: a review. *Curr Diabetes Rev* 2012;8:274-284.

[30] Bloomgarden Z. Screening for and managing diabetic retinopathy: current approaches. *Am J Health Syst Pharm* 2007; 64(17, Suppl. 12): S8-S14.

[31] Ryan G. New pharmacologic approaches to treating diabetic retinopathy. *Am J Health Syst Pharm* 2007; 64(17, Suppl. 12): S15-S21.

[32] Jain A, Collen J, Kaines A, Hubschman JP, Schwartz S. Short-duration focal pattern grid macular photocoagulation for diabeticmacular edema: four-month outcomes. *Retina* 2010; 30:1622-1626.

[33] Sivaprasad S, Elagouz M, McHugh D, Shona O, Dorin G. Micropulsed diode laser therapy: evolution and clinical applications. *Surv Ophthalmol* 2010; 55:516-530.

[34] Aiello LP, Avery RL, Arrigg PG, et al. Vascular endothelial growth factor in ocular fluid of patients with diabetic retinopathy and other retinal disorders. *NEJM* 1994; 331;1480-1487.

[35] Ferrara N, Gerber H, Le Couter J. The biology of VEGF and its receptors. *Nat Med* 2003;9:669-676.

[36] Papadopoulos N, Martin J, Ruan Q, Rafique A, Rosconi M, Shi E, et al. Binding and neutralization of vascular endothelial growth factor (VEGF)

and related ligands by VEGF Trap, ranibizumab and bevacizumab. *Angiogenesis* 2012;15:171-185.

[37] Stewart M. Anti-vascular endothelial growth factor drug treatment of diabetic macular edema: the evolution continues. *Curr Diabetes Rev* 2012; 8:237-246.

[38] Ding J, Wong TY. Current epidemiology of diabetic retinopathy and diabetic macular edema. *Curr Diab Rep* 2012;12: 346-354.

[39] Benarous R, Sasongko MB, Qureshi S, et al. Differential association of serum lipids with diabetic retinopathy and diabetic macular edema. Invest Ophthalmol Vis Sci 2011;52:7464-7469.

[40] Lim LS, Wong TY. Lipids and diabetic retinopathy. *Expert Opin Biol Ther* 2012;12:93-105.

[41] Bhagat N, Grigorian RA, Tutela A, Zarbin MA. Diabetic macular edema: pathogenesis and treatment. *Surv Ophthalmol* 2009;54:1-32.

[42] Bressler NM, Miller KM, Beck RW, et al; for the Diabetic Retinopathy Clinical Research Network. Observational study of subclinical diabetic macular edema. *Eye (Lond)* 2012; 26:833-840.

[43] Mitchell P, Bandello F, Schmidt-Erfurth U, et al; for the RESTORE study group. The RESTORE study: ranibizumab monotherapy or combined with laser versus laser monotherapy for diabetic macular edema. *Ophthalmology* 2011;118: 615-625.

[44] Elman MJ, Aiello LP, Beck RW, et al; for the Diabetic Retinopathy Clinical Research Network. Randomized trial evaluating ranibizumab plus prompt or deferred laser or triamcinolone plus prompt laser for diabetic macular edema. *Ophthalmology* 2010;117:1064-1077.

[45] Elman MJ, Bressler NM, Qin H, et al; for the Diabetic Retinopathy Clinical Research Network. Expanded 2-year followup of ranibizumab plus prompt or deferred laser or triamcinolone plus prompt laser for diabetic macular edema. *Ophthalmology* 2011;118:609-614.

[46] Elman MJ, Qin H, Aiello LP, et al; for the Diabetic Retinopathy Clinical Research Network. Intravitreal ranibizumab for diabetic macular edema with prompt versus deferred laser treatment: three-year randomized trial results. *Ophthalmology* 2012;119:2312-2318.

[47] Ip M, Domalpally A, Hopkins J, Wong P, Ehrlich J. Long-term effects of ranibizumab on diabetic retinopathy severity and progression. *Arch Ophthalmol* 2012;130: 1145-1152.

[48] Rajendram R, Fraser-Bell S, Kaines A, et al. A 2-year prospective randomized controlled trial of intravitreal bevacizumab or laser therapy

(BOLT) in the management of diabetic macular edema: 24-month data: report 3. *Archives of Ophthalmology* 2012;130:972-979.

[49] Macugen 1013 Study Group. A phase 2/3,multicenter, randomized, double-masked, 2-year trial of pegaptanib sodium for the treatment of diabetic macular edema. *Ophthalmology* 2011;118:1107-1118.

[50] RISE and RIDE Research Group. Ranibizumab for diabetic macular edema: results from2 phase iii randomized trials: RISE and RIDE. *Ophthalmology* 2012,119:789-801.

[51] Pan-American Collaborative Retina Study Group (PACORES). Intravitreal bevacizumab plus grid laser photocoagulation or intravitreal bevacizumab or grid laser photocoagulation for diffuse diabetic macular edema: results of the Pan-american Collaborative Retina Study Group at 24 months. *Retina* 2013;33:403-413.

[52] RISE and RIDE Research Group. Ranibizumab for diabetic macular edema: results from2 phase iii randomized trials: RISE and RIDE. *Ophthalmology* 2012;119:789-801.

[53] RESTORE Study Group. The restore study: ranibizumab monotherapy or combined with laser versus laser monotherapy for diabetic macular edema. *Evidence-Based Ophthalmology* 2011;12:206-207.

[54] READ-2 Study Group. Primary end point (six months) results of the ranibizumab for edema of themacula in diabetes (READ-2) study. *Ophthalmology* 2009;116:175-2181.

[55] READ-2 Study Group. Two-year outcomes of the ranibizumab for edema of the macula in diabetes (READ-2) study. *Ophthalmology* 2010;117:2146-2151.

[56] Massin P, Bandello F, Garweg JG, et al. Safety and efficacy of ranibizumab in diabeticmacular edema (RESOLVE study): a 12-month, randomized, controlled, double-masked, multicenter phase II study. *Diabetes Care* 2010;33:2399-2405.

[57] DA VINCI Study Group. One-year outcomes of theDA VINCI study of VEGF trap-eye in eyes with diabetic macular edema. *Ophthalmology* 2012;119:1658-1665.

[58] Diabetic Retinopathy Clinical Research Network. Intravitreal ranibizumab for diabetic macular edema with prompt versus deferred laser treatment: three-year randomized trial results. *Ophthalmology* 2012;119:2312-2318.

[59] Gragoudas E, Adamis A, Cunningham E, Jr, Feinsod M, Guyer D. Pegaptanib for neovascular age-related macular degeneration. *N Engl J Med* 2004;351: 2805-2816.

[60] Ferrara N, Damico L, Shams N, Lowman H, Kim R. Development of ranibizumab, an antivascular endothelial growth factor antigen binding fragment, as therapy for neovascular age-related macular degeneration. *Retina* 2006;26: 859-870.

[61] Yu L, Liang X, Ferrara N. Comparing protein VEGF inhibitors: in vitro biological studies. *Biochem Biophys Res Commun* 2011;408: 276-281.

[62] Holash J, Davis S, Papadopoulos N, Croll S, Ho L, Russell M, et al. VEGF-Trap: a VEGF blocker with potent antitumor effects. *Proc Natl Acad Sci* USA 2002; 99: 11393-11398.

[63] Joussen AM, Poulaki V, Le ML, et al. A central role for inflammation in the pathogenesis of diabetic retinopathy. *The FASEB Journal* 2004; 18:1450-1452.

[64] Diabetic Retinopathy Clinical Research Network. Three-year follow-up of a randomized trial comparing focal/grid photocoagulation and intravitreal triamcinolone for diabetic macular edema. *Arch Ophthalmol* 2009;127:245-251.

[65] Audren F, Lecleire-Collet A, Erginay A, et al. Intravitreal triamcinolone acetonide for diffuse diabetic macular edema: phase 2 trial comparing 4 mg vs 2 mg. *Am J Ophthalmol* 2006;142:794.e8–799.e8.

[66] Gillies MC, Sutter FKP, Simpson JM, Larsson L, Ali H, Zhu M. Intravitreal triamcinolone for refractory diabetic macular edema. Two-year results of a double-masked, placebocontrolled, randomized clinical trial. *Ophthalmology* 2006;113:1533-1538.

[67] Kuppermann BD, Blumenkranz MS, Haller JA, et al. Randomized controlled study of an intravitreous dexamethasone drug delivery system in patients with persistent macular edema. *Arch Ophthalmol* 2007;125:309-317.

[68] Comyn O, Lightman SL, Hykin PG. Corticosteroid intravitreal implants vs. ranibizumab for the treatment of vitreoretinal disease. *Curr Opin Ophthalmol* 2013;24:248-254.

[69] Callanan DG, Jaffe GJ, Martin DF, et al. Treatment of posterior uveitis with a fluocinolone acetonide implant: three-year clinical trial results. *Arch Ophthalmol* 2008; 126:1191-1201.

[70] Alimera Sciences (2013). Alimera Sciences announces ILUVIEN® now available in U.K. Available at: http://investor.alimerasciences.com/releasedetail.cfm?ReleaseID=759915 (accessed 12 September 2013).

[71] Campochiaro P, Brown D, Pearson A, Ciulla T, Boyer D, Holz F, et al. Long-term benefit of sustained-delivery fluocinolone acetonide vitreous

inserts for diabetic macular edema. *Ophthalmology* 2011; 118: 626-635 e2.

[72] Campochiaro P, Brown D, Pearson A, Chen S, Boyer D, Ruiz-Moreno J, et al. Sustained delivery fluocinolone acetonide vitreous inserts provide benefit for at least 3 years in patients with diabetic macular edema. *Ophthalmology* 119: 2125-2132.

[73] Kane FE, Burdan J, Cutino A, Green KE. Iluvien: a new sustained delivery technology for posterior eye disease. *Expert Opin Drug Deliv* 2008; 5:1039-1046.

[74] Pearson PA, Comstock TL, Ip M, et al. Fluocinolone acetonide intravitreal implant for diabetic macular edema: a 3-year multicenter, randomized, controlled clinical trial. *Ophthalmology* 2011;118:1580-1587.

[75] Callanan D, Gupta S, Boyer D, Ciulla T, Singer M, Kuppermann B, et al. Dexamethasone intravitreal implant in combination with laser photocoagulation for the treatment of diffuse diabetic macular edema. *Ophthalmology* 2013;120:1843-1851.

[76] Diabetic Retinopathy Clinical Research Network. Three-year follow-up of a randomized trial comparing focal/grid photocoagulation and intravitreal triamcinolone for diabetic macular edema. *Arch Ophthalmol* 2009;127:245-251.

[77] Campochiaro PA, Hafiz G, Shah SM, et al. Sustained ocular delivery of fluocinolone acetonide by an intravitreal insert. *Ophthalmology* 2010; 117:1393-1399.

[78] Ozurdex CHAMPLAIN Study Group. Dexamethasone intravitreal implant for treatment of diabetic macular edema in vitrectomized patients. *Retina* 2011;915-923.

[79] Gillies MC, McAllister IL, Zhu M, et al. Intravitreal triamcinolone prior to laser treatment of diabetic macular edema: 24-month results of a randomized controlled trial. *Ophthalmology* 2011;118: 866-872.

[80] Gillies MC, Simpson JM, Gaston C, et al. Five-year results of a randomized trial with open-label extension of triamcinolone acetonide for refractory diabetic macular edema. *Ophthalmology* 2009;116:2182-2187.

[81] Yanyali A, Horozoglu F, Celik E, Ercalik Y, Nohutcu AF. Pars plana vitrectomy and removal of the internal limiting membrane in diabetic macular edema unresponsive to grid laser photocoagulation. *Eur J Ophthalmol* 2006;16:573-581.

[82] Thomas D, Bunce C, Moorman C, Laidlaw DA. A randomised controlled feasibility trial of vitrectomy versus laser for diabetic macular oedema. *Br J Ophthalmol* 2005;89:81-86.
[83] Dhingra N, Sahni J, Shipley J, et al. Vitrectomy and internal limiting membrane (ILM) removal for diabetic macular edema in eyes with absent vitreo-macular traction fails to improve visual acuity: results of a 12 months prospective randomized controlled clinical trial. *Invest Ophthalmol Vis Sci* 2005;46:E-Abstract 1467.
[84] Bahadir M, Ertan A, Mertoglu O. Visual acuity comparison of vitrectomy with and without internal limiting membrane removal in the treatment of diabetic macular edema. *Int Ophthalmol* 2005;26:3–8.
[85] Kim YT, Kang SW, Kim SJ, Kim SM, Chung SE. Combination of vitrectomy, IVTA, and laser photocoagulation for diabetic macular edema unresponsive to prior treatments; 3-year results. *GraefesArchClin Exp Ophthalmol* 2012;250:679-684.
[86] Kang SW, Park SC, Cho HY, Kang JH. Triple therapy of vitrectomy, intravitreal triamcinolone, and macular laser photocoagulation for intractable diabetic macular edema. *Am J Ophthalmol* 2007;144:878-885.
[87] Robaszkiewicz J, Chmielewska K, Figurska M, Wierzbowska J, Stankiewicz A. Triple therapy: phaco-vitrectomy with ILM peeling, retinal endophotocoagulation, and intraoperative use of bevacizumab for diffuse diabetic macular edema. *Med Sci Monit* 2012;18:CR241-CR251
[88] Virgili G, Parravano M, Menchini F, Brunetti M. Antiangiogenic therapy with anti-vascular endothelial growth factor modalities for diabetic macular oedema. *Cochrane Database Syst Rev* 2012;12:CD007419.
[89] Wang H, Sun X, Liu K, Xu X. Intravitreal ranibizumab (Lucentis) for the treatment of diabetic macular edema: a systematic review and meta-analysis of randomized clinical control trials. *Curr Eye Res* 2012;37:661-670.
[90] Nguyen QD, Brown DM, Marcus DM, et al; for the RISE and RIDE Research Group. Ranibizumab for diabetic macular edema: results from 2 phase III randomized trials: RISE and RIDE. *Ophthalmology* 2010;119:789-801.
[91] Nguyen QD, Shah SM, Khwaja AA, et al. Two-year outcomes of the ranibizumab for edema of the macula in diabetes (READ-2) study. *Ophthalmology* 2010;117:2146-2151.

[92] Do DV, Nyuyen QD, Khwaja AA, et al. Ranibizumab for edema of the macula in diabetes study. 3-year outcomes and the need for prolonged frequent treatment. *JAMA Ophthalmol* 2013;131:139-145.

[93] Aiello LP, Beck RW, Bressler NM, et al; for the Diabetic Retinopathy Clinical Research Network. Rationale for the diabetic retinopathy clinical research network treatment protocol for center-involved diabetic macular edema. *Ophthalmology* 2011;118:e5-14.

[94] Dowler JG, Hykin PG, Lightman SK, Hamilton AM. Visual acuity following extracapsular cataract extraction in diabetes: a meta-analysis. *Eye (Lond)* 1995;9(Pt 3):313-317.

[95] Soheilian M, Garfami KH, Ramezani A, Yaseri M, Peyman GA. Two-year results of a randomized trial of intravitreal bevacizumab alone or combined with triamcinolone versus laser in diabetic macular edema. *Retina* 2012;32:314-321.

[96] Sultan MB, Zhou D, Loftus J, Dombi T, Ice KS, for the Macugen 1013 Study Group. A phase 2/3, multicenter, randomized, double-masked, 2-year trial of pegaptanib sodium for the treatment of diabetic macular edema. *Ophthalmology* 2011;118:1107-1118.

In: Macular Edema
Editor: Earl Davison
ISBN: 978-1-63321-584-9


*Chapter 5*

# CURRENT MANAGEMENT OF CHRONIC DIABETIC MACULAR OEDEMA

***Will Foulsham[1] and V. Swetha E. Jeganathan[2,3,*]***

[1]Forth Valley Royal Hospital, Larbert, UK
[2]Princess Alexandra Eye Pavillion, Edinburgh, UK
[3]Department of medicine, University of Edinburgh, UK

## ABSTRACT

Diabetic macular oedema (DMO) is a leading cause of visual impairment in people with diabetes mellitus. Defined as retinal thickening involving or approaching the center of the macula, if left untreated more than half of patients lose more than two lines of visual acuity within 2 years. DMO results in a significant socioeconomic burden, particularly affecting the working-age population. This burden will increase in parallel with the inexorable rise in the prevalence of diabetes globally. A thorough understanding of the pathogenesis of chronic DMO is required to delineate the functional and clinical characteristics of the disease. Furthermore, for effective management of the condition, a multidisciplinary approach is necessary with intervention at both systemic and local levels. Treatment for DMO is continuously evolving with the advent of novel pharmacologic therapies. Despite this, focal laser photocoagulation remains the mainstay of

* Correspondence: Dr V.Swetha E. Jeganathan, Princess Alexandra Eye Pavillion, 45 Chalmers Street, Edinburgh EH3 9HA, United Kingdom. Email: vswetha@ausdoctors.net.

treatment. Data from the most recent clinical trials of therapies for this complex condition have confirmed the benefit of intravitreal antivascular endothelial growth factor (anti-VEGF) medications and corticosteroids. The aim of this review is to provide an overview of current treatment perspectives by discussing the various treatment options for chronic DMO.

## INTRODUCTION

Diabetic macular oedema (DMO) is the most common cause of vision loss in patients with diabetic retinopathy [1, 2]. Approximately half of untreated patients with DMO will lose two or more lines of visual acuity within 2 years [3]. Visual loss reduces quality of life for diabetic patients by compromising independence, mobility, self-care and leisure activities [4].

The treatment paradigm for DMO has been in a state of flux over recent years, driven by the development of novel pharmacological agents. In this new era, emphasis on managing the risk factors for development of DMO remains as important as ever. The purpose of this chapter is to give an overview of the current management strategies in DMO and propose a treatment algorithm that will aid clinicians in managing such cases in their clinical practice.

## EPIDEMIOLOGY OF DIABETIC MACULAR OEDEMA

The prevalence of diabetes is predicted to increase globally by more than 50% from 2000 to 2030 [5]. Diabetic retinopathy is the leading cause of preventable blindness in working-age adults in developed countries [6, 7]. In the Wisconsin Epidemiologic Study of Diabetic Retinopathy (WESDR), 3.6% of patients diagnosed with diabetes before the age of 30 and 1.6% of those diagnosed after the age of 30 were legally blind [8]. Diabetic patients perceive blindness to be the third worst complication of their condition, following strokes and amputation [9].

At the time of diagnosis of diabetes, retinopathy is present in up to 30% of individuals [10]. Patients with type 1 diabetes are less likely to have retinopathy at diagnosis (less than 4%), but have higher incidence (approximately 6%) [11, 12]. Indeed, some studies have observed retinopathy being virtually universal in type 1 patients at 20 years follow-up [13]. Klein et al reported the incidence of macular oedema over a 10 year period to be 20.1%

in the younger-onset group, 25.4% in the older-onset group taking insulin, and 13.9% in the older-onset group not taking insulin.

Visual impairment represents a significant cost to the economy through rehabilitation, lost labour force participation, welfare provision, caring services and concessions. [14] The total annual cost of DMO to England is estimated to be in excess of £116 million [15].

The prevalence of DMO is predicted to rise over coming years especially in developed countries. However, some optimism can be gleaned from earlier diagnosis of diabetes, as well as increased emphasis on lifestyle modification and advances in pharmacology. These measures will help control risk factors contributing to DMO. Nevertheless, it is clear that DMO will continue to be a significant burden for both individuals and the wider economy in decades to come.

## Pathophysiology of Chronic Diabetic Macular Oedema

Diabetic maculopathy refers to retinal thickening involving or approaching the center of the macula, and can be further classified as: focal oedema, diffuse oedema, ischaemic or mixed. DMO may be tractional due to vitreoretinal pathology or non-tractional (intraretinal). The pathophysiology of DMO is complex. The common pathway is the breakdown of the blood-retinal barrier (BRB), which results in the accumulation of fluid in retinal tissue. Several factors contribute to the disruption of the BRB, including incompetent tight junctions, loss of endothelial cells, increased vesicular transport, retinal vessel leukostasis and increased permeability of retinal pigment epithelium cells.

The pathogenesis involves the interaction of several systems. Ischemia and inflammation increase the synthesis of vascular endothelial growth factor (VEGF), which is potent stimulant of angiogenesis. Furthermore, VEGF increases vascular permeability through the formation of fenestrations on endothelial cells and the dissolution of tight junctions [16, 17]. Chronic hyperglycaemia results in the accumulation of free radicals, advanced glycation end-products and protein kinase C that further increase the synthesis of VEG-F [18]. Studies demonstrating that strict glycaemic control yields significant clinical benefits support the hypothesis that hyperglycaemia plays a significant role in pathogenesis [19, 20]. The renin-angiotensin-aldosterone system contributes by causing endothelin-mediated vasoconstriction and worsening hypoxia [21].

It has been postulated that the mechanical factors of vitreomacular traction and adhesion may have a role to play in the pathogenesis of DMO. This is corroborated by the observation that the posterior vitreous detachment is less common in eyes with DMO than eyes without [22]. In laboratory investigations, it has been demonstrated that capillary stretching increases VEGF production [23].

## INVESTIGATIONS FOR DMO

Diagnosis of DMO requires careful examination with high magnification, stereoscopic biomicroscopy (e.g., 78D lens). The visual acuity (VA) is best measured with the ETDRS chart, but the Snellen is widely used in clinical practice. Other ancillary investigations such as optical coherence tomography (OCT) can provide important information regarding treatment and follow-up. In particular, the advent of OCT has revolutionised the monitoring of DMO. By reflecting light off retinal structures, OCT creates cross-sectional images of the retina. Figure 1 illustrates an example OCT image in a patient with DMO. These images can provide information about anatomical changes to the retina over time. Having obtained widespread acceptance as a useful modality to assess macular pathology, there are now classification systems based on the location and amount of retinal thickening on OCT assessment. These new classification systems take consideration of parameters such as central retinal thickness, extension of retinal thickening, macular volume, retinal morphology and the existence of vitreo-retinal traction.

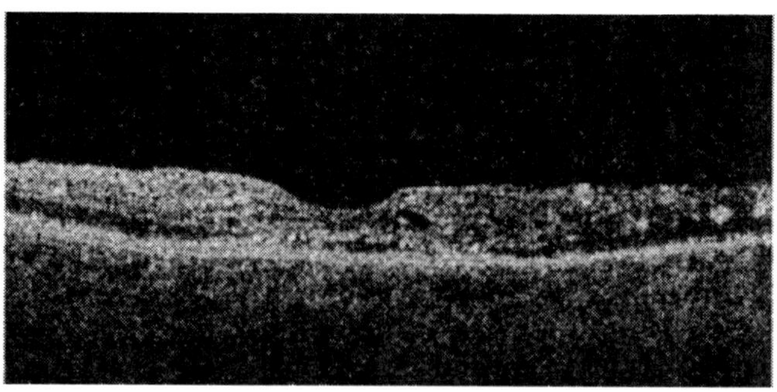

Figure 1. Macula OCT showing diffuse DMO.

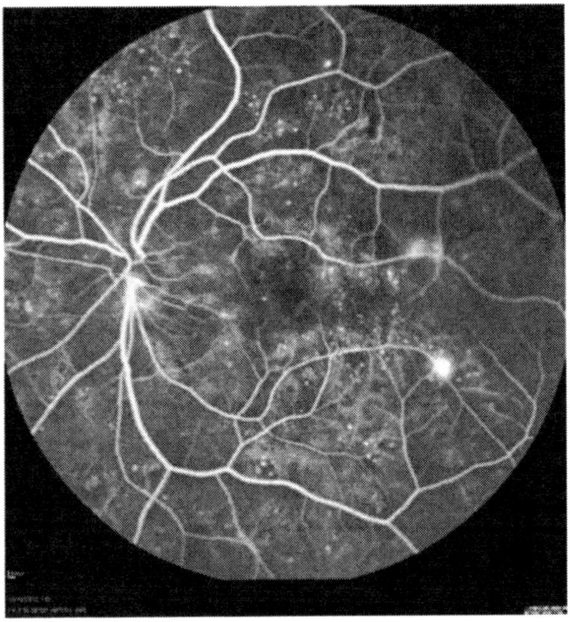

Figure 2. FFA identifying mixed maculopathy.

Fluorescein angiography (FFA) is often used to guide management, especially in distinguishing between focal and diffuse disease. FFA identifies leakage, extent, and macular ischemia. This information also helps determine which type of laser photocoagulation therapy is most appropriate for the patient. Figure 2 provides an example image.

## The Role of Systemic Risk Factors

The risk factors for progression to DMO include duration of DM, hyperglycaemia, hypertension and dyslipidaemia [24, 25, 26, 27]. Studies have shown that hyperglycaemia (measured as glycosylated haemoglobin at initial evaluation) was a strong predictor of incidence and progression of DMO [28]. The United Kingdom Prospective Diabetes Study (UKPDS) has demonstrated the cost-effectiveness and efficacy of optimal glycaemic control in diabetic eye disease [29]. Strict glycaemic control (HbA1c values around 6.5%) is associated with delayed progression of DMO [30]. The UKPDS has also produced evidence that tight blood pressure control significantly reduces the proportion of patients with deterioration of diabetic eye disease [31]. Finally, a significant association of increased LDL levels with DMO has been shown [32]. Other microvascular complications of diabetes (e.g., renal disease) can be used as predictors for retinopathy. Proteinuria and elevated urea/creatinine levels are sound indicators of concurrent eye disease. The importance of these strategies in limiting DMO cannot be overemphasized.

## Laser Treatment in the Management of Chronic Diabetic Macular Oedema

Conducted in 1985, the Early Treatment Diabetic Retinopathy Study (ETDRS) demonstrated that focal or grid laser therapy reduced the risk of moderate visual loss by 50% at three years, compared to observation [33]. Since the study, argon photocoagulation has been the mainstay of treatment for clinically significant macular oedema (CSMO).

ETDRS provided the definitions for standardized communication about DMO, by categorizing DMO based on the appearance of fundal photographs. CSMO is diagnosed if the following features are present [34]: (1) retinal thickening at or within 500µm of the centre of the macula; (2) hard exudates at or within 500µm of the centre of the macula if associated with adjacent retinal thickening; (3) retinal thickening of > 1 disc area any part of which is within 1 disc diameter of the centre of the macula. Focal DMO is defined as well circumscribed areas of leakage with oedema and full/part rings of exudates often surrounding a microaneurysm. Diffuse DMO refers to generalized leakage with oedema. Ischaemic DMO describes the situation in which there is a relatively normal clinical appearance, but macular ischemia on fundus fluorescein angiography and decreased visual acuity.

Focal DMO is managed with focal macular photocoagulation. Leaking aneurysms are treated directly with a 50- to 100- µm diameter spot and an exposure of 0.1 s. In contrast, diffuse DMO is treated with grid pattern laser photocoagulation. In this scenario, burns of 50- to 200- µm in diameter produce a pattern that is spaced equally across the macula. The aim is to promote proliferation of pigment epithelial cells in the retina, causing improved integrity of BRB through the replacement of damaged cells. Of note, high power photocoagulation with decreased exposure time can cause tissue damage with retinal haemorrhages. On the other hand, low power with increased exposure can result in poorly defined lesions that tend to increase in size with time.

There are several disadvantages to laser photocoagulation. The main disadvantage is that although laser therapy can stabilize vision, it offers minimal restoration of visual acuity. Indeed, trials following the ETDRS have demonstrated very small gains (<3 letters) for patients receiving laser monotherapy [35, 36]. Recently there has been some evidence to suggest larger gains are possible on laser monotherapy. In a Diabetic Retinopathy Clinical Research Network randomised control trial comparing laser with intravitreal triamcinolone, 26% of those treated with laser monotherapy gained three or more lines [37]. One possible explanation for this is improved glycaemic control – in the original ETDRS study 40% of participants at an HbA1c in excess of 10% [38].

A further disadvantage is that a subset of patients seems to be refractive to laser photocoagulation; their BCVA worsens despite laser therapy. 12% of patients in the ETDRS study lost more than 15 letters at 3-year follow up [39]. Finally, laser photocoagulation carries the risk of significant side effects. These include visual field changes, worsening of colour vision, contrast sensitivity, impaired night driving, nyctalopia, and dark adaptation [25]. A related problem concerns the enlargement of laser scars following treatment. One study following 191 laser scars in 19 eyes demonstrated increased scar size in 89.5% of cases [40]. These scars can impair visual acuity further.

As a response to the significant side effects associated with the ETDRS laser photocoagulation, other protocols involving reduced radiation exposure have been trialled. An example is the subthreshold diode micropulse laser that limits the damage to ocular tissue. Studies comparing the effectiveness of these two laser photocoagulation protocols have demonstrated similar outcomes with respect to visual acuity and retinal thickness [41, 42].

## Anti-VEGF Therapies

Intraocular injections of VEGF antagonists have transformed the management of age-related macular degeneration (AMD) [43]. These therapies are causing a similar paradigm shift in the management of DMO. Indeed, NICE published guidelines in April 2013 recommending ranibizumab (Luncentis, Genentech/Roche) for treatment of DMO when central retinal thickness exceeds 400μm at the start of treatment [44].

The initial loading phase of monthly injections is for 4 to 6 months, followed by PRN phase with continued treatment until the macula is dry or until there is no further improvement. We recommend monthly follow-up of patients undergoing anti-VEGF treatment with OCT scan and visual acuity assessment is required to decide on retreatments. If the patient has been stable off treatment for several monthly assessments, in year 2 onwards the period between follow-up appointments may be increased gradually, ultimately to a maximum of 12- 16 weeks as long as there are no other features requiring more frequent follow-up. Patients unwilling or unsuitable for injections should be offered macular laser treatment if appropriate.

VEGF has been studied in the context of diabetic retinopathy for the past two decades. Initial studies demonstrated that VEGF levels were elevated in cases of diabetic retinopathy [45, 46]. Following this, experimental elevation of VEGF in preclinical studies was demonstrated to induce diabetic retinopathy [47]. In further preclinical models, the VEGF inhibitor pegaptanib (Macugen, Eyetech Pharmaceuticals/Pfizer) was effective in inhibiting both neovascularization and BRB disruption occurring in diabetic retinopathy [48, 49].

Ranibizumab is a fully humanized monoclonal antibody fragment that was designed specifically for use in the eye. Further investigational anti-VEGF therapies include pegaptanib, aflibercept (Regeneron/Bayer HealthCare) and bevacizumab (Avastin, Genentech/Roch). In this chapter, we will review current evidence for the use of ranibizumab in DMO and summarize the studies conducted with alternative anti-VEGF therapies.

A series of RCTs have demonstrated the safety of efficacy of ranibizumab in the treatment of DMO, as well as improved clinical outcomes over laser and IVTA. READ-2 compared three treatment arms; ranibizumab alone, laser alone, and ranibizumab in combination with laser [50]. At 6 months follow-up, there was a significant improvement in best-corrected visual acuity (BCVA) in the ranibizumab alone treatment arm, compared with either laser alone or laser in combination with ranibizumab. REVEAL compared the same treatment arms with a larger study size [51]. At 12 months follow-up, both ranibizumab treatment arms demonstrated a significant improvement in BCVA over laser. The ranibizumab combination therapy with laser was not superior to ranibizumab alone.

Over the past three years, four phase II or III trials (RESOLVE, RESTORE, RISE and RIDE) have shown ranibizumab to be more effective than either sham or laser photocoagulation in both improving BCVA and reducing central retinal thickness (CRT). In RESOLVE, ranibizumab was administered in three monthly injections and then as needed [52]. At 12 months, ranibizumab patients had a mean average increase of BCVA of 7.8 ETDRS letters, whereas sham recipients had a mean decrease of 0.1 letters. Of note, the effect of treatment in the ranibizumab arm was noted at the first follow-up visit (day 8) [45].

In the RESTORE study, a similar treatment pattern of three monthly injections then as needed was followed [53]. Similar groups as the READ-2 study were employed (ranibizumab alone, laser alone and ranibizumab plus laser). At 12 months, ranibizumab therapy demonstrated improved mean BCVA. Adjunctive laser therapy did not show a statistically significant benefit [46]. At 24 months, the results remained consistent [54].

The RISE and RIDE studies compared three study arms; 0.3mg ranibizumab, 0.5 ranibizumab and sham [55, 56]. The greatest gains in BCVA at 24 months in the RISE study belonged to the 0.3mg groups (as measured by proportion of patients with letter gain of greater than 15 ETDRS letters). However, in the RIDE study the 0.5mg group demonstrated the greatest improvement in BCVA. In both RISE and RIDE, the improvement in mean BCVA was significantly greater in either ranibizumab arm than in sham recipients.

In the DRCR.net-1 trial, the four treatment arms were: (1) ranibizumab plus prompt (within 3-10 days post ranibizumab), (2) ranibizumab plus deferred (>24 weeks) laser, (3) triamcinolone plus prompt laser and (4) prompt laser [57]. At 12 months, both functional and anatomical outcomes in the ranibizumab groups (but not triamcinolone plus prompt laser) were greater than prompt laser alone. Notably, ranibizumab with prompt laser therapy had similar efficacy to ranibizumab with delayed laser therapy [58].

The evidence demonstrates that ranibizumab is more effective than laser photocoagulation in the treatment of CSMO. However, it is by no means a panacea. The RISE and RIDE studies illustrate that there is a subgroup of patients with refractory DMO [48], [49]. Indeed, 25% of the 0.3mg ranibizumab group had central foveal thickness greater than 250μm on optical coherence tomography following therapy [59].

The cost of ranibizumab is considerable at $2000 per dose [60]. Alternative VEGF inhibitors are being assessed for efficacy and safety in DMO. For example, bevacizumab is a full-length monoclonal antibody related to ranibizumab that was developed for colorectal cancer. At a cost of $50 per dose, this drug has been widely adopted for off-label use in neovascular ophthalmologic conditions [62]. Indeed, despite its off-label status bevacizumab constitutes the majority of intravitreal anti-VEGF injections around the world. Indeed, in the US, bevacizumab accounts for 58% of all infections for neovascular AMD via fee-for-service Medicare claims [62]. Another treatment option is the VEGF Trap-Eye, a fusion protein consisting of the fragment cystallizable region of IgG human IgG fused with parts of VEGF receptors. One-year outcomes of the DME and VEGF Trap-Eye: Investigation of Clinical Impact (DA VINCI) demonstrate significant gains in BCVA in all VEGF Trap-Eye groups from baseline achieved at week 24 of the study, and maintained to week 52 [63]. The potential advantage of VEGF Trap-Eye is an increased affinity for VEGF-A, resulting in a stable and inert 1:1 complex that requires less frequent dosing [64].

Data regarding the long-term safety profiles of ranibizumab can be extracted from neovascular age-related macular degeneration (AMD) trials. At 24 months' follow-up in the SECURE study, assessing the long-term safety of ranibizumab 0.5mg in exudative wet AMD, the most frequent ocular adverse events were retinal haemorrhage (12.8%), cataract (11.5%) and increased intraocular pressure (6.4%) [65]. In a meta-analysis of ranibizumab trial data intravitreal ranibizumab was associated with an increased incidence of cerebrovascular accidents compared to sham injections (2.2% vs. 0.7% respectively) [66]. This raises concerns for VEGF antagonism in general [67]. The most frequent ocular adverse events in the DA VINCI trial of VEGF Trap-Eye were conjunctival haemorrhage, ocular hyperemia, eye pain and increased intraocular pressure. The final point to emphasize is that VEGF plays several physiological roles in the eye – the long-term sequelae of antagonism have not yet been studied [6].

## Intravitreal Steroids to Treat Chronic Diabetic Macular Oedema

Prior to the development of VEGF antagonists, the synthetic glucocorticoid triamcinolone was the principal intravitreal agent used in the treatment of DMO [68]. Proposed mechanisms of action for triamcinolone include upregulation of production of tight junction proteins between endothelial cells, as well as inhibition of VEGF [69, 70]. By these mechanisms, triamcinolone decreases vessel leakage and promotes angiostasis. Since the early 1990s, preclinical studies have supported the use of intravitreal triamcinolone in DMO by demonstrating inhibition of ocular neovascularization and dampening of the inflammatory cascade [71]. The clinical utility of intravitreal steroid use was further supported by a 2006 RCT of 69 eyes with refractory DMO [72]. At 24 months follow up, visual acuity improvements of five or more letters were seen in 56% of the triamcinolone treatment arm, while only 26% of the placebo arm shared this improvement.

More recently, larger studies have demonstrated inferior clinical outcomes intravitreal triamcinolone monotherapy compared to laser photocoagulation. The DRCR.net 3 year study compared 1mg and 4mg intravitreal triamcinolone with laser therapy in 840 eyes in 693 subjects [73]. At 4 months, the 4mg triamcinolone group demonstrated greater improvements in visual acuity than either of the two other groups. However, this improvement was not maintained. At 2 years, the mean VA was statistically better in the laser photocoagulation group than in the steroid-injected groups. Furthermore, when anatomical changes to the retina were accessed using OCT, the results were consistent with the clinical outcomes.

The DRCR.net study also highlighted the significant adverse effects of intravitreal steroids. Cataract surgery was required in 51% and 23% of the triamcinolone 4mg and 1mg groups, respectively, compared with 13% of patients in the laser photocoagulation arm [64]. Elevated intraocular pressure requiring medication was 12% in the triamcinolone 4mg group, compared with 3% in the laser group.

In another DRCR.net study pseudophakic eyes had superior visual acuity improvements compared to phakic eyes [30]. Indeed, the 62 pseudophakic eyes studied demonstrated improvement comparable to either of the two ranibizumab study groups, and significantly greater improvements than the sham plus prompt laser group. Intravitreal glucocorticoid therapy may still have a role in cases of refractive DMO [74, 75]. Importantly, intravitreal steroids do not appear to be retinotoxic in these patients [76].

Researchers have been keen to establish whether triamcinolone may have a role to play in a combination therapy with either laser photocoagulation. Whilst some studies suggested that combined treatment results in superior outcomes to laser therapy alone [77, 78], others found this effect either non-existent or short-lived [79, 80]. There are RCTs on-going in which triamcinolone is combined with either ranibizumab or bevacizumab. Researchers are interested in whether triamcinolone might reduce the frequency with which VEGF antagonists need to be delivered.

Sustained release devices for delivering intravitreal steroids may help to limit systemic adverse effects, by targeting delivery of the therapeutic agent to the posterior segment. Fluocinolone acetonide intravitreal inserts have been developed that can be implanted into the vitreous cavity via a 25-gauge needle. These inserts have been designed to release a daily dose of either 0.2 or 0.5 μg. Improved visual acuity in DMO at 12 months has been demonstrated in a pharmacokinetic study, in which the device was also shown to deliver consistent dosing for at least 1 year [81]. In a multicentre RCT, patients with DMO refractive to laser photocoagulation were randomised to either 0.2μg fluocinolone acetonide intravitreal insert, 0.5μg insert or sham injection treatment groups. These patients were followed over 24 months. The visual acuity improvements measured by mean improvements in letter score were 5.4, 4.4 and 1.7 letters in the 0.5μg insert, 0.2μg insert and sham injection groups respectively [82]. Although effective at reducing the occurrence of nonocular adverse events, the study groups treated with glucocorticoid therapy are associated with increased incidence of ocular adverse events. Indeed, in the fluocinolone acetonide RCT, increased intraocular pressure requiring surgery occurred in 7.6%, 3.7% and 0.5% of the high-dose, low-dose and sham treatment arms respectively.

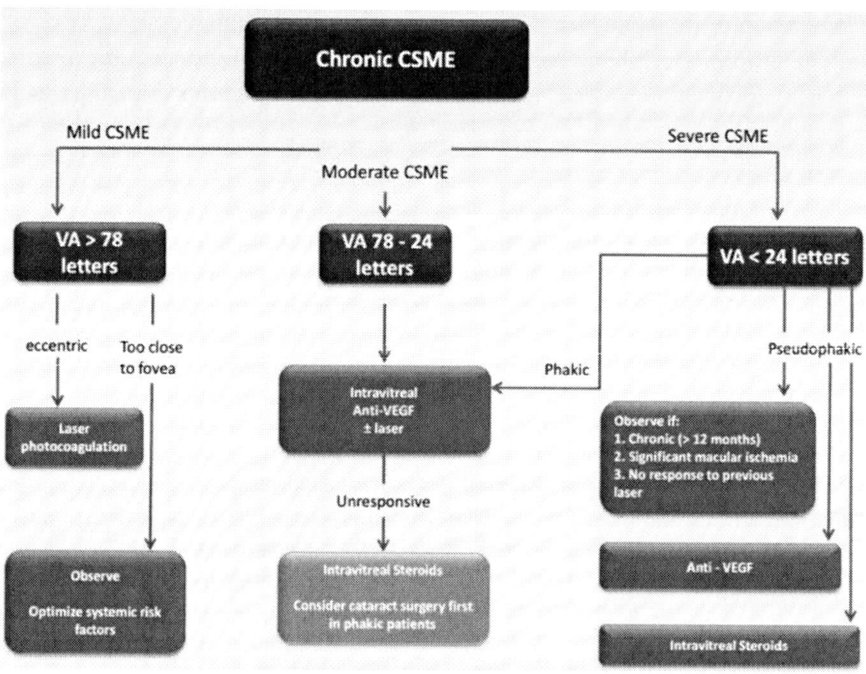


Figure 3. Treatment algorithm for chronic DMO.

# DMO TREATMENT ALGORITHM

## The Treatment of DMO Can Be Challenging

Potential treatment options should be discussed with the patient and treatment should be tailored to meet the individual patient. Some patients may choose different treatment options depending on their circumstances; e.g., some with relatively good vision who feel they are managing well, may choose not to be treated with intravitreal injections. There should be close attention to systemic factors for all cases. We provide a treatment algorithm for chronic DMO based on current consensus of evidence that will aid clinicians managing such cases (Figure 3).

## The Role of Vitrectomy

The vitreous has been described as contributing factor to development of DMO [83]. This is supported by observational evidence that the prevalence of posterior vitreous detachment is lower in eyes with DMO than in eyes without DMO [25]. Further studies showed spontaneous resolution of DMO in 55% of cases with posterior vitreous detachment, compared with 25% of cases with posterior vitreous adhesion [84]. Capillary stretching has been shown to increase thymidine uptake and VEGF production [26]. The contribution of epiretinal tensile forces to the pathogenesis of DMO may help us to understand the subgroup of patients who fail to respond to VEGF antagonist therapy [52].

Since the early 1990s, surgeons have been conducting vitrectomies to treat DMO in patients with evident vitreomacular traction on OCT [85]. Two main theories explain why vitrectomy may be helpful. The mechanical release theory postulates that there is an accumulation of intravitreal chemoattractants following the breakdown of the BRB, which then induce cellular migration at the posterior hyaloid [78]. In turn these cells contract, mediating vitreomacular traction.

The chemical diffusion theory proposes that an incompetent BRB results in the accumulation of growth factors under the premacular posterior hyaloid [86]. Vitrectomy allows the preretinal growth factors to be washed out, and promotes the diffusion of VEGF, IGF-1 and histamines away from the retina [87]. In support of this theory, there is evidence to suggest that victrectomy is effective in resolving DMO in eyes *without* vitreomacular traction [88].

Related to this theory is the proposition is improved transvitreal oxygenation of the retina plays a role [89].

The success of vitrectomy for both functional and anatomical improvements has been demonstrated in a number of retrospective studies [90, 91, 92]. A significant decrease in retinal thickness postoperatively has been found within 1 week of surgery, with a continued decrease up to 4 months [93].

The role of internal limiting membrane (ILM) peeling remains controversial. ILM specimens from eyes with DMO have been shown to be several times thicker than normal ILM, and to contain increased levels of laminin, fibronectin and collagen [94, 95]. These anatomical differences may contribute towards an altered fluid balance between the vitreous and retina. A further suggested mechanism describes a posterior precortical vitreous pocket lying in front of the posterior retina, and extending to the temporal vascular arcades [96]. In performing a posterior vitreous detachment during vitrectomy, only the anterior surface of this pocket would be removed, since the posterior surface is attached to the ILM. It is posited that the posterior surface would continue to exert tractional forces. Numerous small studies have shown improved outcomes with ILM peeling [97]. However, larger studies have demonstrated no improvement in visual acuity despite improved anatomy [98].

There are features of the ILM peeling procedure that potentially compromise visual acuity. Firstly, ILM swelling can result in damage to the adjacent Muller cell endfeet, which can in turn affect the electrophysiological output of the retina. In addition, using stains such as indocyanine green to stain the ILM can have a negative effect on visual function [99]. The physical and chemical insults to the retina during the ILM pealing procedure may help explain the discrepancy between anatomical and functional results.

There are numerous potential adverse events associated with victrectomy, several of which are sight-threatening. In a review of 336 eyes, the incidence of complications was: cataract 11%, retinal tears 9%, development of epiretinal membranes 7%, vitreous haemorrhage 7%, retinal detachment 2%, neovascular glaucoma 2% and macular hole 1% [100].

Vitreomacular traction has been shown to play a role in the development of DMO. In a subset of patients with severe DMO or DMO that is refractive to pharmacologic and laser therapy, we can expect surgical vitrectomy to continue to be a valuable management option.

# FUTURE MANAGEMENT OPTIONS

The incessant rise in the prevalence of DM has prompted researchers to explore new avenues for the management of DMO. There are a number of potentially pathogenic biochemical pathways triggered by hyperglycaemia in the retina, and researchers are evaluating agents that inhibit these pathways [101]. Of particular interest is the polyol pathway, overactivation of which results in increased concentrations of sorbitol and reactive oxygen species, as well as decreased concentrations of nitric acid and glutathione. Sorbitol may glycate nitrogens on certain proteins, resulting in the formation of advanced glycation end-products (AGEs). The activation of receptors for AGEs causes inflammation. It has been demonstrated clinically that inhibiting AGE formation can attenuate DMO [102]. Novel agents to inhibit AGE formation and block AGE receptors are being developed [103].

Studies suggest that PKCβ is an important controller of endothelial cell permeability, and may also have a role in upregulating VEGF [104]. Ruboxistaurin is a PKCβ-isoform inhibitor that aims to reduce retinal permeability and ischaemia-induced neovascularization. In a randomized placebo-controlled trial, exposure to ruboxistaurin resulted in a significantly lower risk of moderate visual loss at six years [105]. Other trials have been less encouraging; the PKC-DMES study found that ruboxistaurin did not have a significant effect on the progression of DMO [106].

The key advantage of topical administration is the avoidance of adverse events associated with intravitreal injection, such as endophthalmitis. Several topical agents for DMO are being investigated. The nicotinic acetylcholine receptor antagonist mecamyalmine has been shown to inhibit angiogenesis at vascular endothelial cells and decrease vascular permeability in animal models [107]. A multicentre phase I/II clinical trial determined that mecamylamine had heterogeneous effects in patients with diabetic macular edema, possibly due to variable expression of nACh subtypes [108]. Nepafenac is a prodrug that is hydrolysed by uveal tissue and the retina to its active form amfenac [109]. A case series of patients treated with nepafenac monotherapy twice daily indicated that the therapy might be beneficial in the treatment of DMO [110]. Further research on these therapies is required.

## Conclusion

Chronic DMO is a major cause of vision loss in patients with diabetes and is associated with a large socioeconomic burden. Anti-VEGF treatments have heralded a new paradigm for the treatment of DMO. However, not all patients are suitable for anti-VEGF treatment and treatment must be individualised. As our understanding of the pathogenesis of DMO deepens, the potential for novel treatments increases. This is reflected in the promise of drugs that modulate the polyol pathway, as well as PKCβ-isoform inhibitors such as roboxistaurin. In our enthusiasm with novel strategies, we must not forget the importance of holistic preventative strategies such as strict glycaemic control and controlling systemic risk factors, which will ultimately save patients' lives.

## References

[1] Frampton JE. Ranibizumab: in diabetic macular oedema. *Drugs* 2012 Mar 5; 72 (4): 509-23.

[2] Nguyen QD, Shah SM, Heier JS, et al. Primary end point (six months) results of the Ranibizumab for Edema of the mAcula in diabetes (READ-2) study. *Ophthalmology* 2009 Nov; 116 (11): 2175-81.e1.

[3] Ferris FL III, Patz A. Macular edema: a complication of diabetic retinopathy. *Surv. Ophthalmol.* 1984; 28 (Suppl.): 452–461.

[4] Coyne KS, Margolis MK, Kennedy-Martina T et al. The impact of diabetic retinopathy: perspectives from patient focus groups. *Family Practice* 2004; 21 (4): 447-453.

[5] Wild S, Roglic G, Green A, et al. Global prevalence of diabetes: estimates for the year 2000 and projections for 2030. *Diabetes Care* 2004;27: 1047-53.

[6] Cheung N, Mitchell P, Wong TY. Diabetic retinopathy. *Lancet* 2010 Jul 10; 376 (9735): 124-36.

[7] NG Congdon, DS Friedman, T Lietman. Important causes of visual impairment in the world today. *JAMA* 2003 Oct 15; 290 (15): 2057-2060.

[8] Klein R, Klein BE, Moss SE, et al. The Wisconsin epidemiologic study of diabetic retinopathy. IV. Diabetic macular edema. *Ophthalmology* 1984; 91:1464-74.

[9] Williams R, Airey M, Baxter H, et al. Epidemiology of diabetic retinopathy and macular oedema: a systematic review. *Eye* (London) 2004;18:963–83.

[10] Williams R, Airey M, Baxter H, et al. Epidemiology of diabetic retinopathy and macular oedema: a systematic review. *Eye* (London) 2004; 18: 963–83.

[11] Frank RN, Hoffman WH, Podgor MJ, Joondeph HC, Lewis RA, Margherio RR et al. Retinopathy in juvenile-onset diabetes of short duration. *Ophthalmology* 1980; 87: 1–9.

[12] Klein R, Palta M, Allen C, Shen G, Han DP, D'Alessio DJ. Incidence of retinopathy and associated risk factors from time of diagnosis of insulin-dependent diabetes. *Arch. Ophthalmol.* 1997; 115: 351–356.

[13] Orchard TJ, Dorman JS, Maser RE, Becker DJ, Drash AL, Ellis D et al. Prevalence of complications in IDDM by sex and duration. Pittsburgh Epidemiology of Diabetes Complications Study II. *Diabetes* 1990; 39: 1116–1124.

[14] Meads C, Hyde C. What is the cost of blindness? *Br. J. Ophthalmology* 2003; 87: 1201-1204.

[15] Minassian DC, Owens DR, Reidy A. Prevalence of diabetic macular oedema and related health and social care resource use in England. *Br. J. Ophthalmol.* 2012; 96: 345–9.

[16] Roberts WG, Palade GE. Increased microvascular permeability and endothelial fenestration induced by vascular endothelial growth factor. *J. Cell Sci.* 1995; 108 (pt6): 2369-79.

[17] Antonetti DA, Khin S , Lieth E, et al., and the Penn State Retina research Group. Vascular permeability in cxperimental diabetes is associated with reduced endothelial occludin content: vascular endothelial growth factor decreases occludin in retinal endothelial cells. *Diabetes* 1998; 47 (12): 1953-9.

[18] Robero-Aroca, P. Targeting the Pathophysiology of Diabetic Macular Edema. *Diabetes Care* 2010; 33 (1): 2484-2485.

[19] Diabetes Control and Complications Trial Research Group. The effect of intensive treatment of diabetes on the development and progression of long-term complications in insulin-dependent diabetes mellitus. *N. Engl. J. Med.* 1993; 329 (14): 977-86.

[20] Diabetes Control and Complications Trial Research Group. Progression of retinopathy with intensive versus conventional treatment in the Diabetes Control and Complications Trial. *Ophthalmology* 1995; 102(4): 647-61.

[21] Jeganathan VS. The therapeutic implications of renin-angiotensin system blockade in diabetic retinopathy. *Curr. Pharm. Biotechnol.* 2011 Mar 1;12 (3): 392-5.

[22] Nasrallah FP, Jalkh AE, Coppenolle FV, Kado M, Trempe CL, McMeel JW, et al. The role of the vitreous in diabetic macular edema. *Opthalmology*. 1988; 95: 1335-1339.

[23] Seko Y, Seko Y, Fujikura H, Pang J, Tokoro T, Shimokawa H. Induction of vascular endothelial growth factor after application of mechanical stress to retinal pigment epithelium of the rat in vitro. *Invest. Ophthalmol. Vis. Sci.* 1999; 40:3287-3291.

[24] Klein R, Knudtson MD, Lee KE, et al. The Wisconsin Epidemiologic Study of Diabetic Retinopathy XXIII: the twenty-five-year incidence of macular edema in persons with type 1 diabetes. *Ophthalmology* 2009; 116: 497–503.

[25] Knudsen LL, Lervang HH, Lundbye-Christensen S, et al. The North Jutland County Diabetic Retinopathy Study (NCDRS) 2. Non-ophthalmic parameters and clinically significant macular oedema. *Br. J. Ophthalmol.* 2007; 91: 1593–5.

[26] Kamoi K, Takeda K, Hashimoto K, Tanaka R, Okuyama S. Identifying risk factors for clinically significant diabetic macula edema in patients with type 2 diabetes mellitus. *Curr. Diabetes Rev.* 2013 May; 9 (3): 209-17.

[27] Diep TM, Tsui I. Risk factors associated with diabetic macular edema. *Diabetes Research and Clinical Practice* 2013 June; 100 (3): 298-305.

[28] Klein R, Klein BEK, Moss SE, Davis MD, DeMets DL. Glycosylated hemoglobin predicts the incidence and progression of diabetic retinopathy. *JAMA* 1988; 260 (19): 2864-71.

[29] UK Prospective Diabetes Study Group. Intensive blood-glucose control with sulphonylureas or insulin compared with conventional treatment and risk of complications in patients with types 2 diabetes (UKPDS 33). *Lancet* 1998; 352: 837-53.

[30] Mohamed Q, Gillies MC, Wong TY; Management of diabetic retinopathy: a systematic review. *JAMA*. 2007 Aug 22; 298 (8): 902-16.

[31] UK Prospective Diabetes Study Group. Tight blood pressure control and risk of macrovascular and microvascular complications in type 2 diabetes: UKPDS 38. *BMJ* 1998; 317 (7160): 703-713.

[32] Idiculla J, Nithyanandam S, Joseph M, Mohan VKA et al. Serum lipids and diabetic retiniopathy: A cross-sectional study. *Indian Journal of Endocrinology and Metabolism* 2012; 16 (8): 492-494.

[33] Early photocoagulation for diabetic retinopathy. ETDRS report number 9. Early Treatment Diabetic Retinopathy Study Research Group. *Ophthalmology* 1991; 98: 766-85.

[34] Early Treatment Diabetic Retinopathy Study Research Group: Photocoagulation for diabetic macular edema. ETDRS report No 4. *Int. Ophthalmol. Clin.* 1987; 27: 254-264.

[35] Mitchell P, Bandello F, Schmidt-Erfurth U, Lang GE, Massin P, Schlingermann RO et al. The RESTORE study: ranibizumab monotherapy or combined with laser versus laser monotherapy for diabetic macular edema. *Ophthalmology* 2011; 118: 615-625.

[36] Elman MJ, Aiello LP, Beck RW, Bressler NM, Bressler SB, Edwards AR et al. Randomized trial evaluating ranibizumab plus prompt or deferred laser or triamcinolone plus prompt laser for diabetic macular edema. *Ophthalmology* 2010; 117: 1064-1077.

[37] Beck RW, Edwards AR, Aiello LP et al. Three-year follow-up of a randomized trial comparing focal/grid photocoagulation and intravitreal triamcinolone for diabetic macular edema. *Arch. Ophthalmol.* 2009; 127: 245-51.

[38] Williams MA, Chakravarthy U. Evidence underlying the clinical management of diabetic macular oedema. *Clinical Medicine* 2013; 13 (4): 353-7.

[39] Photocoagulation for diabetic macular edema. Early Treatment Diabetic Retinopathy Study report number 1. Early Treatment Diabetic Retinopathy Study research group. *Arch. Ophthalmol.* 1985; 103: 1796-1806.

[40] Maeshima K, Utsugi-Sutoh N, Otani T, et al. Progressive enlargement of scattered photocoagulation scars in diabetic retinopathy. *Retina* 2004; 24(4): 507-11.

[41] Figueira J, Khan J, Nunes S, et al. Prospective randomized controlled trial comparing sub-threshold micropulse diode laser photocoagulation and conventional green laser for clinically significant diabetic macular oedema. *Br. J. Ophthalmol.* 2009; 93 (10): 1341-4.

[42] Vujosevic S, Bottega E, Casciano M, et al. Microperimetry and fundus autofluorescence in diabetic macular edema: subthreshold micropulse diode laser versus modified early treatment diabetic retinopathy study laser photocoagulation. *Retina* 2010; 30 (6): 908-16.

[43] Jeganathan Vs. Anti-angiogenesis drugs in diabetic retinopathy. *Curr. Pharm. Biotechnol.* 2011 Mar; 12 (3): 369-72.

[44] National Institute for Clinical Excellence. TA274 Ranibizumab for treatment diabetic macular oedema (rapid review of technology appraisal guidance 237). http://publications.nice.org.uk/ranibizumab-for-treating-diabetic-macular-oedema-rapid-review-of-technology-appraisal-guidance-ta274/guidance (accessed 10th June 2014).

[45] Aiello LP, Avery RL, Arrigg PG, et al. Vascular endothelial growth factor in ocular fluid of patients with diabetic retinopathy and other retinal disorders. *N. Engl. J. Med.* 1994; 331 (22): 1480-7.

[46] Adamis AP, Miller JW, Bernal MT, et al. Increased vascular endothelial growth factor levels in the vitreous of eyes with proliferative diabetic retinopathy. *Am. J. Ophthalmol.* 1994; 118 (4): 445-50.

[47] Tolentino MJ, Miller JW, Gragoudas ES, et al. Intravitreous injections of vascular endothelial growth factor produce retinal ischemia and microangiopathy in an adult primate. *Opthalmology* 1996; 103 (11): 1820-8.

[48] Ishida S, Usui T, Yamashiro K, et al. VEGF164 is proinflammatory in the diabetic retina. *Invest. Ophthalmol. Vis. Sci.* 2003; 44 (5): 2155-62.

[49] Ishida S, Usui T, Yamashiro K, et al. VEGF164-mediated inflammation is required for pathological, but not physiological, ischemia-induced retinal neovascularization. *J. Exp. Med.* 2003; 198 (3): 483-9.

[50] Nguyen QD, Shah SM, Khwaja AA, et al. Two-year outcomes of the ranibizumab for edema of the mAcula in diabetes (READ-2) study. *Ophthalmology* 2010; 117: 2146–51.

[51] Ohji M, Ishibashi T Sr, REVEAL study group. Efficacy and safety of ranibizumab 0.5 mg as monotherapy or adjunctive to laser versus laser monotherapy in Asian patients with visual impairment due to diabetic macular edema: 12-month results of the REVEAL Study [abstract]. *Invest. Ophthalmol. Vis. Sci.* 2012; 53: E-Abstract 4664.

[52] Massin P, Bandello F, Garweg JG, et al. Safety and efficacy of ranibizumab in diabetic macular edema (RESOLVE study): a 12-month, randomized, controlled, double-masked, multicentre phase II study. *Diabetes Care* 2010 Nov; 33 (11): 2399-405.

[53] Mitchell P, Bandello F, Schmidt-Erfurth U, et al. The RESTORE study: ranibizumab monotherapy or combined with laser versus laser monotherapy for diabetic macular edema. *Ophthalmology* 2011; 118 (4): 615-625.

[54] Mitchell P, RESTORE extension study group. 2-Year safety and efficacy outcome of ranibizumab 0.5 mg in patients with visual impairment due to diabetic macular edema (DME): an interim analysis

of the RESTORE extension study [abstract]. *Invest. Ophthalmol. Vis. Sci.* 2012; 53: E-Abstract 4667.

[55] Genentech. A study of ranibizumab injection in subjects with clinically significant macular edema with center involvement secondary to diabetes mellitus (RIDE) [Clinical-Trials.gov identifier NCT00473382]. US National Institutes of Health, ClinicalTrials.gov [online]. Available from URL: http://clinicaltrials.gov (accessed 9th June 2014)

[56] Boyer DS, Sy J, Chen Rundle A, et al. Ranibizumab (anti-VEGF) for vision loss due to diabetic macular edema: rsults of two phase III randomized trials [abstract 0132-LBOR]. 71st Annual Scientific Sessions of the American Diabetes Association; 2011 June 24-28; San Diego (CA)

[57] Diabetic Retinopathy Clinical Research Network, Elman MJ, Bressler NM, et al. Expanded 2-year follow-up of ranibizumab plus prompt or deferred laser or triamcinolone plus prompt laser for diabetic macular edema. *Ophthalmology* 2011 Apr; 118 (4): 609-14.

[58] Diabetic Retinopathy Clinical Research Network, Elman MJ, Aiello LP, et al. Randomized trial evaluating ranibizumab plus prompt or deferred laser or triamcinolone plus prompt laser for diabetic macular edema. *Ophthalmology* 2010 Jun; 117 (6): 1064-77.e35.

[59] Telander D, Hunter A. The evolving paradigm for the treatment of diabetic macular edema. *Ophthalmic Surgery, Lasers and Imaging Retina* 2013 Jul; 44 (4): 324-328.

[60] Nwanze CC, Akinwale A, Adelman RA. Bevacizumab vs. Ranibizumab in preserving or improving vision in patients with wet, age-related macular degeneration: a cost-effectiveness review. *Clin. Med. Insights: Ther.* 2012; 4:29–38.

[61] Jackson TL, Kirkpatrick L. Cost comparison of ranibizumab and bevacizumab. *BMJ* 2011; 343: d5058.

[62] Brechner RJ, Rosenfeld PJ, Babish JD, Caplan S. Pharmacotherapy for neovascular age-related macular degeneration: an analysis of the 100% 2008 Medicare fee-for-service part B claims file. *Am. J. Ophth.* 2011; 151 (5): 887-895.

[63] Do DV, Nguyen QD, Boyer D et al. One-year outcomes of the da Vinci Study of VEGF Trap-Eye in eyes with diabetic macular edema. *Ophthalmology*. 2012 Aug; 119 (8): 1658-65.

[64] Rudge JS, Holash J, Hylton D, et al. Inaugural Article: VEGF Trap complex formation measures production rates of VEGF, providing a

biomarker for predicting efficacious angiogenic blockade. *Proc. Natl. Acad. Sci. USA*. 2007; 104: 18363-18370.

[65] Silva R, Axer-Siegel R, Eldem B, Guymer R. The SECURE study: long-term safety of ranibizumab 0.5mg in neovascular age-related macular degeneration. *Ophthalmology*. 2013 Jan; 120 (1): 130-9.

[66] Ueta T, Yanagi Y, Tamaki Y, et al. Cerebrovascular accidents in ranibizumab [letter]. *Ophthalmology* 2009; 116 (2): 362.

[67] Lim LS, Cheung CM, Mitchell P, Wong TY. Emerging evidence concerning systemic safety of anti-VEGF agents – should ophthalmologists be concerned? *Am. J. Ophthalmol.* 2011 Sep; 152 (3): 329-31.

[68] Cunningham MA, Edelman JL, Kaushal S. Intravitreal steroids for macular edema: the past, the present and the future. *Surv. Ophthalmol.* 2008; 53 (2): 139-49.

[69] Sears JE, Hoppe G. Triamcinolone acetonide destabilizes VEGF mRNA in muller cells under continuous cobalt stimulation. *Invest. Ophthalmol. Vis. Sci.* 2005; 46: 4336-4341.

[70] Gardner TW, Antonetti DA, Barber AJ et al; Penn State Retina Research Group. Diabetic retinopathy: more than meets the eye. *Surv. Ophthalmol.* 2000; 47 (Supp): S253-S262.

[71] Danis RP, Bingaman DP, Yang Y, et al. Inhibition of preretinal and optic nerve head neovascularization in pigs by intravitreal triamcinolone acetonide. *Ophthalmology* 1996; 103 (12): 2099-104.

[72] Gillies MC, Sutter FK, Simpson JM, et al. Intravitreal triamcinolone for refractory diabetic macular edema: tow-year results of a double-masked, placebo-controlled, randomized clinical trial. *Ophthalmology* 2006; 113 (9): 1533-8.

[73] Beck RW, Edwards AR, Aiello LP, et al. Three-year follow-up of a randomized trial comparing focal/grid photocoagulation and intravitreal triamcinolone for diabetic macular edema. *Arch. Ophthalmol.* 2009; 127: 245-251.

[74] Martidis A, Duker JS, Greenberg PB et al. Intravitreal triamcinolone for refractory diabetic macular edema. *Ophthalmology* 2002; 109: 920-927.

[75] Massin P, Audren F, Haouchine B et al. Intravitreal triamcinolone acetonide for diabetic diffuse macular edema: preliminary results of a prospective controlled trial. *Ophthalmology* 2004; 111: 218-225.

[76] Lang Y, Leibu R, Shoham N et al. Evaluation of intravitreal Kenalog toxicity in humans. *Ophthalmology* 2007; 114: 724-731.

[77] Lam DS, Chan CK, Mohamed S, et al. Intravitreal triamcinolone plus sequential grid laser versus triamcinolone or laser alone for treating diabetic macular edema: six-month outcomes. *Ophthalmology* 2007; 114 (12): 2162-7.

[78] Maia Jr OO, Takahashi BS, Costa RA et al. Combined laser and intravitreal triamcinolone for proliferative diabetic retinopathy and macular edema: one-year results of a randomized clinical trial. *Am. J. Ophthalmol.* 2009; 147 (2): 291-7.

[79] Lee HY, Lee SY, Park JS. Comparison of photocoagulation with combined intravitreal triamcinolone for diabetic macular edema. *Korean J. Ophthalmol.* 2009; 23 (3): 153-8.

[80] Mirshahi A, Shenazandi H, Lashay A, et al. Intravitreal triamcinolone as an adjunct to standard laser therapy in coexisting high-risk proliferative diabetic retinopathy and clinically significant macular edema. *Retina* 2010; 30 (2): 254-9.

[81] Campochiaro PA, Hafiz G, Shah SM et al. Famous study group. Sustained ocular delivery of fluocinolone acetonide by an intravitreal insert. *Ophthalmology* 2010; 117: 1393-1399.

[82] Campochiaro PA, Brown DM, Pearson A et al. Long-term benefit of sustained-delivery fluocinolone acetonide vitreous inserts for diabetic macular edema. *Ophthalmology* 2011; 118: 626-635.

[83] Nasrallah FP, Van De Velde F, Jalk AE et al. Importance of the vitreous in young diabetic with macular edema. *Ophthalmology* 1989; 96: 1511-1516.

[84] Hikichi T, Fugio N, Akidba J, Azuma Y, Tadabashi M, Yashida A. Association between the short term natural history of diabetic macular edema and the vitreomacular relationship in Type 2 diabetes mellitus. *Ophthalmology* 1997; 104: 473-478.

[85] Lewis H, Abrams GW, Blumenkranz MS, Camp RV. Vitrectomy for diabetic macular traction and edema associated with posterior hyaloidal traction. *Ophthalmology* 1992; 99 (5): 753-759.

[86] Stolba U, Binder S, Gruber D, Krebs I, Aggermann T, Neumaier B. Vitrectomy for persistent diffuse diabetic macular edema. *Am. J. Ophthalmol.* 2005; 140 (2): 295-301.

[87] Meyer CH. Current treatment approaches in diabetic macular edema. *Ophthalmologica* 2007; 221: 118-31.

[88] La Heij EC, Hebdrikse F, Kessels AGH, Derhaag PJ. Vitrectomy results in diabetic macular oedema without evident vitreomacular traction. *Graefes Ach. Clin. Exp. Ophthalmol.* 2001; 239 (4): 264-270.

[89] Stefansson E. Ocular oxygenation and the treatment of diabetic retinopathy. *Surv. Ophthalmol.* 2006; 51 (4): 364-380.

[90] Harbour JW, Smiddy WE, Flynn HW Jr, Rubsamen PE. Vitrectomy for diabetic macular edema associated with a thickened and taut posterior hyaloid membrane. *Am. J. Ophthalmol.* 1996; 121: 405-413.

[91] Pendergast SD: Vitrectomy for diabetic macular edema associated with a taut premacular posterior hyaloid. *Curr. Opin. Ophthalmol.* 1998; 9: 71-75.

[92] Kaiser PK, Riemann CD, Sears JE, Lewis H: Macular traction detachment and diabetic macular edema associated with posterior hyaloidal traction. *Am. J. Ophthalmol.* 2001; 131: 44-49.

[93] Horle S, Poestgens H, Schmidt J, Kroll P: Effect of pars plana vitrectomy for proliferative diabetic vitreoretinopathy on preexisting diabetic maculopathy. *Graefe's Arch. Clin. Exp. Ophthalmol.* 2002; 240:197-201.

[94] Matsunaga N, Ozeki H, Hirabayashi Y, Shimada S, Ogura Y. Histopathologic evaluation of the internal limiting membrane surgically excised from eyes with diabetic maculopathy. *Retinal* 2005; 25, 311-316.

[95] Kohno T, Sorgente N, Doodnight R, Ryan SJ. Alterations in the distribution of fibronectin and laminin in the diabetic human eye. *Invest. Ophthalmol. Vis. Sci.* 1987; 28: 515-521.

[96] Kishi S, Shimizu K: Posterior vitreous precortical pocket. *Arch. Ophthalmol.* 1990; 108: 979-982.

[97] Hartley KL, Smiddy WE, Flynn HW Jr, Murray TG. Pars plana vitrectomy with internal limiting membrane peeling for diabetic macular edema. *Retina*. 2008; 28 (3): 410-419.

[98] Diabetic Retinopathy Clinical Research Network Writing Committee on behalf of the DRCR.net; Haller JA, Qin H, Apte RS et al. Vitrectomy outcomes in eyes with diabetic macular edema and vitreomacular traction. *Ophthalmology* 2010; 117: 1087-1093.

[99] Rodrigues EB, Meyer CH, Farah ME, Kroll P: Surgical management of epiretinal membrane with indocyanine-green-assisted peeling. *Ophthalmologica* 2004; 218: 73-74.

[100] Christoforidis JB, D'Amico DJ. Surgical and other treatments of diabetic macular edema: an update. *Int. Ophthalmol. Clin.* 2004; 44 (1): 139-60.

[101] Curtis TM, Gardiner TA, Stitt AW. Microvascular lesions of diabetic retinopathy: clues towards understanding pathogenesis? *Eye* (Lond). 2009 Jul; 23 (7): 1496-508.

[102] Bolton WK, Cattran DC, William ME, et al. Randomized trial of an inhibitor of formation of advanced glycation end products in diabetic nephropathy. *Am. J. Nephrol.* 2004 Jan; 24 (1): 32-40.

[103] Jeganathan VS. Novel pharmacotherapies for diabetic retinopathy: current and future perspectives. *Curr. Pharm. Biotechnol.* 2011; 12 (3): 336.

[104] Xu X, Qi Z, Xin X, Zhang S, Gu Q, Luo D. Blood-retinal barrier breakdown induced by activation of protein kinase C via vascular endothelial growth factor in streptozotocin-induced diabetic rates. *Curr. Eye Res.* 28, 251-256 (2004).

[105] Lorenzi M. The polyol pathway as a mechanism for diabetic retinopathy: attractive, elusive, and resilient. *Experimental diabetes research* 2007; 2007: 61038.

[106] The PKC-DMES Study Group. Effect of ruboxistaurin in patients with diabetic macular edema: thirty-month results of the randomized PKC-DMES clinical trial. *Arch. Ophthalmol.* 2007: 125 (3), 318-324.

[107] Kiuchi K, Matsuoka M, Wu JC et al. Mecamylamine suppresses basal and nicotine-stimulated choroidal neovascularization. *Invest. Ophthalmol. Vis. Sci.* 49, 1705-1711 (2008).

[108] Campochiaro PA, Shah SM, Hafiz G et al. Topical mecamylamine for diabetic macular edema. *Am. J. Ophthalmol.* 2010 May; 149 (5): 839-51.

[109] Ke TL, Graff G, Spellman JM, Yanni JM. Nepafenac, a unique nonsteroidal prodrug with potential utility in the treatment of trauma-induced ocular inflammation: II. In vitro bioactivation and permeation of external ocular barriers. *Inflammation.* 2000 Aug; 24(4):371-84.

[110] Callanan D, Williams P. Topical nepafenac in the treatment of diabetic macular edema. *Clin. Ophthalmol.* 2008 Dec; 2 (4): 689-692.

In: Macular Edema
Editor: Earl Davison

ISBN: 978-1-63321-584-9


*Chapter 6*

# MACULAR EDEMA IN IMPORTANT TROPICAL INFECTIONS

***Beuy Joob[1] and Viroj Wiwanitkit[2]***
[1]Sanitation 1 Medical Academic Center
[2]Hainan Medical University, China;
Faculty of Medicine, University of Nis, Serbia

## ABSTRACT

There are many problematic tropical infections at present. The good examples include dengue, malaria, etc. Those infections can have the ophthalmological presentations. The ophthalmological presentations might be difficult to diagnose and easily forgotten. This might bring several unwanted outcome. The macular edema is a serious eye disorder that can be seen in many conditions including to the tropical infections. In this specific short article, the authors summarize on important tropical infections and the relating problems of macular edema. The discussion will cover the risk, treatment, complication and outcome of those macular edema disorders in present clinical practice.

**Keywords:** Macular, edema, tropical infection

# Introduction [1 - 3]

There are many problematic tropical infections at present. The good examples include dengue, malaria, etc. Those infections can have the ophthalmological presentations. The ophthalmological presentations might be difficult to diagnose and easily forgotten [1 – 3]. In the cases that the problems occur in the traveler, it might be underdiagnosed in their hometown [4]. This might bring several unwanted outcome.

The macular edema is a serious eye disorder that can be seen in many conditions including to the tropical infections. In this specific short article, the authors summarize on important tropical infections and the relating problems of macular edema. The discussion will cover the risk, treatment, complication and outcome of those macular edema disorders in present clinical practice.

# Macular Edema in Some Important Tropical Infections

1. Malaria

   Malaria is an important tropical parasitic infection. It is caused by pathogenic Plasmodium spp. This infection is a mosquito borne infectious disease that is common in tropical zone. The patients usually present high fever and might have other associated clinical manifestations. The ocular presentation in malaria is very interesting [5]. Focusing on macular edema, there are some reports on this problem among the patients with malaria. According to a recent report from Malawi by White et al., it is concluded that "cerebral malaria was distinguished by sequestration of parasitized erythrocytes, the presence and severity of retinal hemorrhages, the presence of cystoid macular edema [6]." In fact, the macular edema is an important post-fever retinal complication in malaria to be concerned [7]. The great risk is among the patients with severe malaria especially for those with cerebral malaria. The standard treatment of maculopathy is recommended and the result is not different from general cases with macular edema problem.
2. Dengue

   Dengue is another important tropical borne infection. It can be seen in many tropical countries. This infection has a classical presentation of acute febrile illness with hemorrhagic complication. The eye problem in dengue can also be seen [8]. Macular involvement can be observable [8]. Wen et al. noted that "the ocular fundus changes included macular hemorrhage, retinal hemorrhage, maculopathy, Roth's spot, diffuse retinal edema, peripapillary hemorrhage vitreous cells and blurring optic disc [9]." As noted macular edema is an important ocular complication in dengue [10]. The great risk is among the patients with dengue shock. Focusing on the pathogenesis, it is suggested that the macular edema in dengue might be an immune-mediate pathology. The standard treatment of maculopathy is recommended. Nah et al. noted that the problem can have self-resolving with good prognosis [11]. Nah et al. also noted that "treatment is controversial, but a course of corticosteroids has been tried in view of a postulated underlying immune-mediated pathology [11]." For the prognosis, Teoh et al. noted that "the visual outcome was independent of the extent of edema, but scotomata persisted longest in patients with foveolitis and shortest with those with diffuse retinal thickening [12]."

3. Chikungunya

   Chikungunya is another important tropical borne infection that has clinical similarity to dengue but less hemorrhagic complication. The macular edema is also an important post-fever retinal complication in Chikungunya to be concerned [7]. The standard treatment of maculopathy is recommended and the result is not different from general cases with macular edema problem.

4. Cysticercosis

   Cysticercosis is an important tropical cestode infestation. This is a tissue parasitic infestation and the lesion can be seen in any tissue of human body including in eye tissue. The ocular cysticercosis is sporadically reported. Focusing on macular edemia in cysticerosis, there are some interesting reports. Subretinal cyst associated with macular edema can be seen [13]. Besada et al. noted that "ocular signs of disk edema and macular serous fluid secondary to neurocysticercosis may correspond to optic nerve, parenchymal, or extraparenchymal disease [14]." For management of cysticercosis, the surgical removal of the parasite is usually the recommended effective therapeutic choice.

# Conclusion

Macular edema is an important eye problem that can be seen in many tropical infections. The practitioner has to concern on this problem and this should be a caution for any patients living or having history of travel to tropical area.

# References


[1] Johnson, GJ. The environment and the eye. *Eye (Lond)*. 2004 Dec, 18(12), 1235-50

[2] Nentwich, MM; Schaller, UC; Klauss, V. Update, diagnosis and therapy of tropical diseases - part 1. *Klin Monbl Augenheilkd*. 2009 Sep, 226(9), R139-5

[3] Maurin, JF; Renard, JP; Ahmedou, O; Bidaux, F; Dordain, Y; Pariselle, J; Froussart, F; Dot, C; Rigal-Sastourne, JC. Corneal blindness in tropical areas. *Med Trop (Mars)*. 1995, 55(4 Pt 2), 445-9.

[4] Leggat, PA; Speare, R; Moon, ME. Sore eyes and travelers. *J Travel Med*. 1999 Mar, 6(1), 45-7.

[5] Abramson, J; Kushnick, HJ; Mayers, M. Ocular manifestations of systemic infection. *Curr Opin Ophthalmol*. 1994 Dec, 5(6), 84-90.

[6] White, VA; Lewallen, S; Beare, NA; Molyneux, ME; Taylor, TE. Retinal pathology of pediatric cerebral malaria in Malawi. *PLoS One*. 2009, 4(1), e4317.

[7] Vishwanath, S; Badami, K; Sriprakash, KS; Sujatha, BL; Shashidhar, SD; Shilpa, YD. Post-fever retinitis, a single center experience from south India. *Int Ophthalmol*. 2013 Dec 21. [Epub ahead of print]

[8] Lim, WK; Mathur, R; Koh, A; Yeoh, R; Chee, SP. Ocular manifestations of dengue fever. *Ophthalmology*. 2004 Nov, 111(11), 2057-64.

[9] Wen, KH; Sheu, MM; Chung, CB; Wang, HZ; Chen, CW. The ocular fundus findings in dengue fever. *Gaoxiong Yi Xue Ke Xue Za Zhi*. 1989 Jan, 5(1), 24-30

[10] Tan, CS; Teoh, SC; Chan, DP; Wong, IB; Lim, TH. Dengue retinopathy manifesting with bilateral vasculitis and macular oedema. *Eye (Lond)*. 2007 Jun, 21(6), 875-7.

[11] Nah, G; Tan, M; Teoh, S; Chong, CH. Maculopathy associated with Dengue fever in a military pilot. *Aviat Space Environ Med.* 2007 Nov, 78(11), 1064-7.

[12] Teoh, SC; Chee, CK; Laude, A; Goh, KY; Barkham, T; Ang, BS; Eye Institute Dengue-related Ophthalmic Complications Workgroup. Optical coherence tomography patterns as predictors of visual outcome in dengue-related maculopathy. *Retina.* 2010 Mar, 30(3), 390-8.

[13] Bartholowmew, RS. Subretinal cysticercosis. *Am J Ophthalmol.* 1975 Apr, 79(4), 670-3.

[14] Besada, E; Barr, R; Natu, A. Bilateral disk edema with unilateral macular serous fluid secondary to neurocysticercosis. *Optometry.* 2005 Apr, 76(4), 239-49.

In: Macular Edema
Editor: Earl Davison

ISBN: 978-1-63321-584-9


*Chapter 7*

# CYSTOID MACULAR EDEMA: A DIFFICULT OCULAR DISORDER TO CURE

*W. Burke*[1,2,*]
[1]Brain Research Laboratory, Discipline of Physiology, and Bosch Institute, University of Sydney, Australia
[2]Discipline of Anatomy and Histology, University of Sydney, Australia

## ABSTRACT

This article is concerned with the problem of treating cystoid macular edema. The various methods of treating macular edema are briefly described and then a case report on a patient, the author, is presented.

The author developed cystoid macular edema following an operation to cure a macular hole by vitrectomy. Four treatments were applied. All were successful to some degree but none abolished the edema. Details of two treatments, anti-inflammatory eye-drops and acetazolamide (a carbonic anhydrase inhibitor), will not be presented. The other two treatments, hyperbaric oxygen and estrogen, are described in moderate detail and the reason why macular edema is so difficult to treat is discussed in some detail. Suggestions are made as to how the research should proceed.

* Corresponding author: address for correspondence: Prof. W. Burke, Discipline of Physiology, Anderson Stuart Building (F13), University of Sydney, NSW 2006, Australia. Phone: 61 2 9351 6547, Fax: 61 2 9351 2058, Email: william.burke@sydney.edu.au

**Keywords:** Macular edema, hyperbaric oxygen, estrogen, blood-retina barrier, tight junctions

## INTRODUCTION

Macular edema is created in several ways. It can result from cataract surgery, uveitis, diabetic neuropathy, age-related macular degeneration and virtually any inflammatory condition of the eye. Like edema elsewhere in the body it consists of excess fluid both extracellular and intracellular. It is generally agreed that it eventually results in a breakdown of the blood-retina barrier (BRB). The BRB is a double layer of cells, the inner layer being the capillary endothelial cells joined to each other by tight junctions, the outer layer being the retinal pigment epithelial cells, also hound to each other by tight junctions. The presence of the excess fluid distorts the image on the photoreceptor layer and so impairs vision, but there is also a disturbance of metabolism which may cause loss of cells. The vitreous humor filling the posterior chamber and covering the retina is considered to have a protective function, even though its removal does not stop the retina working reasonably well.

## MACULAR HOLE

The vitreous is in close contact with the retina but with injury and certain ocular diseases it may detach. As mentioned earlier, the retina will function without the vitreous but an injury may cause the retina to detach from the pigment epithelium and this will destroy function in the detached part of the retina. This is because the photoreceptor photopsins can only regenerate with the help of the pigment epithelium. In the elderly the vitreous tends to shrink and to pull away from the retina but it is more closely attached at the macula than at the more peripheral parts of the retina, and so tends to pull on the retina, often breaking the junction of retina and pigment epithelium. If this is not treated, the retina is lost in the detached region and leaves a circular 'hole' (a macular hole). The standard treatment is now a vitrectomy. If done quickly and efficiently, good vision is preserved. Unfortunately, even if vision is restored, macular edema may develop. The reason for this is uncertain.

# TREATMENT OF MACULAR EDEMA

For reasons that are not fully understood the various ways of treating macular edema have mixed results. Some patients respond well, others don't. The main methods that have been used are: anti-inflammatory drugs, carbonic anhydrase inhibitors, laser photocoagulation, restoration of the BRB.

## Anti-Inflammatory Drugs

Intraocular inflammation involves the release of prostaglandins, which tend to cause the disruption of the tight junctions in the capillaries, so weakening the BRB and causing edema. Nonsteroidal anti-inflammatory drugs (NSAIDS) act by inhibiting the enzyme cyclooxygenase which is involved in the creation of the prostaglandins. A well-known NSAID is ketorolac tromethamine.

## Steroidal Drugs

Some steroids, e.g., corticosteroids, are also anti-inflammatory, inhibiting the enzyme phospholipase A2 , which is involved in the creation of both prostaglandins and leucotrienes. Leucotrienes are a major cause of inflammation in several regions. Another steroid used to inhibit inflammation in the eye is prednisolone (Pediapred). This acts in a more complex way by gene suppression. Triamcinolone acetonide (several trade names) is a corticosteroid used to treat many diseases, including macular edema. It is usually administered by injection into the vitreous from which it is slowly released. It acts both as an anti-inflammatory and to repair the BRB.

## Carbonic Anhydrase Inhibitors

Carbonic anhydrase (CA) is the enzyme in many regions of the body, but especially the lungs and kidney, that catalyses the conversion of carbon dioxide to carbonic acid. It is therefore of prime metabolic importance. CA also catalyses the reverse equation, creating carbon dioxide from bicarbonate but at a much slower rate. Therefore, inhibitors of CA tend to cause accumulation and then excretion of bicarbonate, accompanying cations (mainly sodium) and water. This acidifies the blood and tissue fluid, causing hyperventilation, thus increasing blood levels of oxygen and decreasing levels of carbon dioxide. This, in turn, lowers the blood pressure and intraocular pressure. Reduction in the intraocular pressure reduces the edema and so is also a favourable treatment for glaucoma. Acetazolamide (Diamox) is a popular and effective CA inhibitor.

## Laser Photocoagultion

This technique is to cauterize leaking ocular blood vessels on a micro scale and also to discourage angiogenesis.

## Hyperbaric Oxygen (HBO)

The rationale for using increased levels of oxygen is the belief that macular edema is due to a state of hypoxia in the retina. Oxygen in high concentration has been used in the study of physiology for a long time [1]. Its effect on vision has been slight except for its effect on premature infants. Premature babies develop a retinopathy involving a delayed development and misdirection of blood vessels (retinopathy of prematurity) and this condition is exaggerated by high oxygen, e.g., 75% [2]. In the 1930s the navies of the U.S.A. and Britain used HBO to treat decompression sickness (the 'bends') [3]. During the second world war several divers in the British Navy experienced blindness or convulsions when they breathed HBO, probably because it was administered at too high a pressure or for too long. These may have been the earliest victims of oxygen toxicity. The study of the toxicity of oxygen at concentrations above normal pressure was commenced in the 1950s [4].

There is also evidence that HBO is effective in repairing a fault in the BRB. Chang and colleagues [5], using streptozotocin-induced diabetic rats, showed that the permeability of the BRB in these rats was decreased by HBO.

There are few reports relating to the application of HBO to ocular diseases. Although there were several reports in the 1960s (refs 6,7,8) the effects were weak and not always in agreement. In 2002 Krott and colleagues [9] used HBO to treat patients with macular edema. The results were confused because retinal photocoagulation was necessary in most cases. No morphological improvement was found in diabetic patients, while in patients with retinal vein occlusions the edema was reduced. In 2004 Jansen & Nielsen [10] used HBO to treat 2 patients experiencing chronic cystoid macular edema but who were refractory to other treatments. Each patient was given 5 daily treatments of 90 minutes at 2.4 atmospheres pressure. Both patients improved rapidly and with long-lasting results (> 7 months). Visual acuity was restored to almost normal and the edema disappeared.

There are several problems in the use of HBO therapy. A general risk is the possibility of convulsion, although all hyperbaric chambers are now monitored with great care. There are usually limits of pressure at 3 atmospheres and duration of 2 hours. Similarly, ophthalmic side-effects are usually avoided by careful monitoring. Myopia may occur but is always reversible. The most serious effect is the creation or exacerbation of cataract but this may be partly reversible.

## Case Report

I wish to report my acquisition of a macular edema and my experiences trying to cure this condition, unsuccessfully as it happened. At the age of about 79 years a macular edema arose in my left eye subsequent to a vitrectomy to cure a macular hole. The operation was completely successful but within a few weeks the edema developed. At first, this was treated with anti-inflammatory eye-drops, but soon I switched to acetazolamide (Diamox, Sigma). Acetazolamide reduced the edema and improved the visual acuity but did not restore normal conditions, so after about two years I discontinued this treatment. This drug is well known for treating macular edema and in many patients it works in a completely satisfactory way, so I don't need to say anything more about it. A year or two later I switched to HBO. At this time the appearance of the edema was similar to that shown in Figure 1.

### Measurement of Visual Acuity

For the purposes of this treatment I used a method of measuring visual acuity intended to obtain the acuity in distinct parts of the macula. The method is fully described in a previous paper [11]. Briefly, the procedure is as follows. I place my head in an ophthalmology head rest, positioned so that my eye is a fixed distance from the screen of a computer monitor. Normally this distance is 57 cm, so that 1 cm on the screen subtends an angle of 1°.

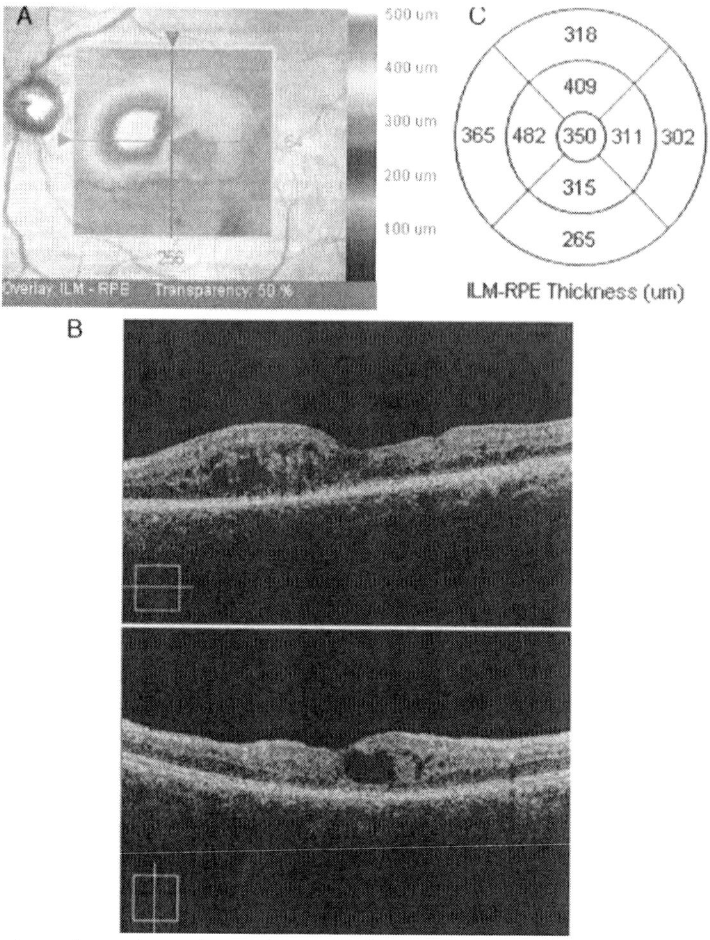


A. Plan view of macula to show edema, thickness of retina colored according to scale on right. B. Transectional views of macula, horizontal on upper; vertical on lower. C. Diagram of macula to show the retinal thickness in the different regions.

Figure 1. Optical coherence tomography (OCT) records from Zeiss OCT Scanner.

On the screen is displayed a St Andrew's cross, but in which the cross-bars do not extend to the centre. The field of view is divided into 9 areas similar to those in the plan of the macula as shown in Figure 1. In each test run I focus on the place where the cross-bars would meet if extended. This is the point of focus. My right eye is covered. A letter can be flashed in any of the 9 areas. The flash lasts 100ms i.e. less than the reaction time. The initial letter flashed in any area has a size of ~1cm x 1cm, i.e. ~1° x 1°.

The flash is triggered by pressing the space bar. I tap the letter key that I think correctly identifies the flashed letter. If I identify correctly, when a letter is flashed in the same area the next time, its size is reduced by a factor of $\sqrt{2}$. Otherwise the size remains unchanged. Fourteen different letters were used. The particular letter and the area in which it was flashed were varied randomly. Eventually, by increasing or decreasing the size of the letters, for each area the size of the letter that I could recognise correctly on 75% of trials was determined. This value is therefore a threshold: the lower the letter size the higher the acuity.

## Measurement of Macula Thickness

The retina was examined with the Optical Coherence Tomography technique (OCT: Carl Zeiss Meditec, Inc). Examples of the transverse radial sections and plan views of the macula are shown in Figure 1. The retina thickness is calculated automatically by the Zeiss instrument and, for each of the 9 sections of the macula, is displayed on the circular graph.

## Treatment with HBO

My treatment with hyperbaric oxygen was conducted in the Diving and Hyperbaric Department of the Prince of Wales Hospital, Sydney, New South Wales, Australia. The sessions took place in a multiplace chamber seating up to fifteen seated patients. The gas used was 100% oxygen at a pressure of 2.4 atmospheres and for a duration of 2 hours, followed by 30 minutes transition to room air at normal pressure. I had 16 sessions extending over three weeks (see Figure 2). Immediately after each session I determined my visual acuity. Whenever possible, the retina was examined with a Zeiss OCT machine but this could not be done as often as with the acuity measurements. Figure 2 illustrates the time courses of the changes in visual acuity at one area of the retina (upper outer fovea) and of the retinal thicknesses in the same region. This region was chosen because it was not a total scotoma and so the acuity could be measured and it could vary according to treatment and other conditions. Under the influence of the HBO the visual acuity altered within a day or two and resumed the control value in less than a week. Retinal thickness probably follows a similar time course, although an inadequate number of records were obtained at the end of the experiment. It was clear that the HBO had a definite effect on both visual acuity and on the macular edema but also that there was no lasting effect. There did not seem to be any point in pursuing the HBO treatment.

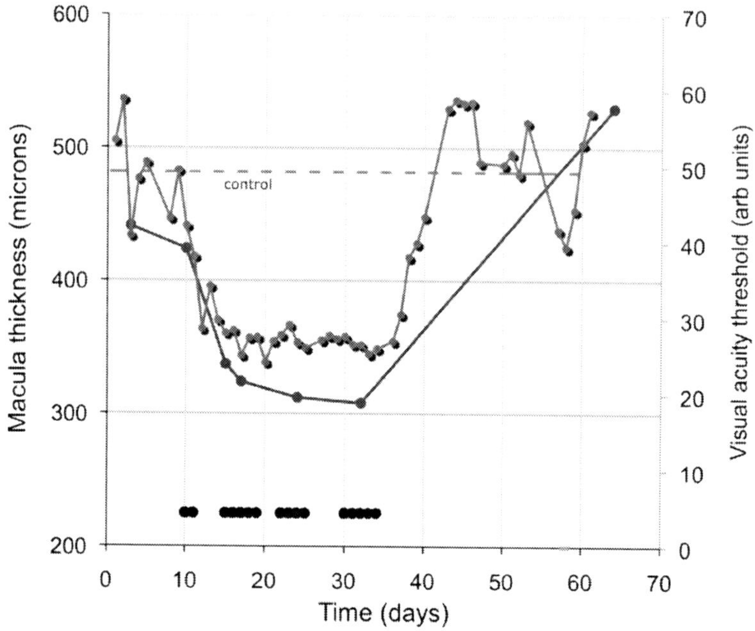


Figure2. Effect of hyperbaric oxygen on macula thickness and visual acuity. The visual acuity thresholds are shown in red, the macula thicknesses in blue. Each black symbol represents an HBO session.

## Treatment with Estrogen

It is known that estrogen protects against stroke by reducing edema, at least partly by reducing the Na-K-Cl co-transporter activity in the blood-brain barrier [12]. The blood-retina barrier (BRB) is regarded as similar to, and perhaps identical with, the blood-brain barrier, and therefore there is a strong possibility that estrogen would reduce macular edema and increase visual acuity.

Accordingly, I applied estradiol glucuronide (Sigma Aldrich) eye drops 4 times a day over a period of about 6 weeks. Figure 3 is a graph of the visual acuity records. The estradiol salt was dissolved in normal saline and the concentration was varied from 5 μg/ml (first 3 records), to 50μg/ml (2 records), to 0.5mg/ml (10 records), then back to 50μg/ml (2 records) and 5μg/ml (2 records The weakest concentration (the first 5 records) probably has no effect, but the next 10 records (0.5mg/ml) show a clear decrease in acuity threshold. With a return to the weaker concentrations and discontinuance of the eye drops, the acuity threshold moves back to the control level. These records resemble those obtained with HBO.

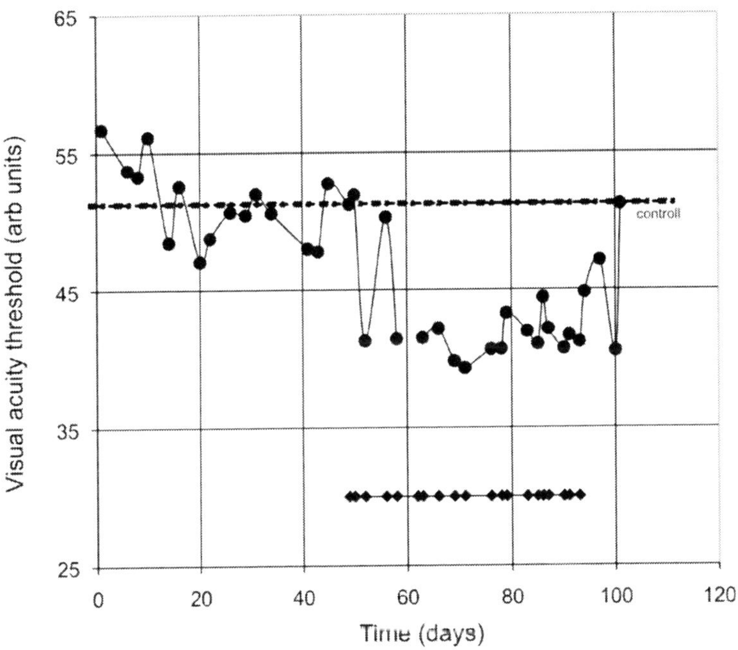


Figure 3. Effect of estradiol on visual acuity. The round black symbols are the visual acuity thresholds. The black diamonds indicate the days on which estradiol eye drops, four times a day, were administered. Further details in text.

There is a clear reduction in acuity threshold occurring within a day or two, well maintained during the procedure but failing within a few days of the return to normal conditions.

On another occasion I studied the effect on my visual acuity of applying estradiol patches (50μg and 100 μg) to my skin, but these had no effect. There are other examples where estrogen patches have been much less effective than when the estrogen is applied orally or parenterally (e.g., Pfaffenrath [13].)

## Discussion

The results from using HBO in my case were disappointing when compared with those obtained by Jansen and Nielsen[10] who obtained good results lasting more than 7 months. It's possible that the difference between their results and mine may have been due to their different etiologies. One of their two patients had type 2 diabetes, the other a complicated cystoid maculopathy. There does not seem to have been a confirmation of Jansen and Nielsen's findings.

I am not aware of estrogen being used to treat macular edema, but obviously this is a method that should be studied in more detail.

There are many treatments for macular edema and most of them are effective to some degree, yet complete cures are often unobtainable. There may be several reasons for this. The first reason is that there may be several independent causes, as mentioned in the Introduction to this chapter. For this reason a treatment may remove one cause but not another. Secondly, a disease affecting several organs in the body may progress if the fundamental cause of the disease is not eliminated. A good example of such a disease is diabetes. Lastly, other events occurring in life may complicate the treatment. For example, because my macular hole was treated by a vitrectomy, my macular edema could not be treated by intravitreal triamcinolone because the slow-release effect due to the vitreous was lost.

I am unable to say precisely why both the HBO and the estrogen became effetive and then ceased to be effective so quickly, but the most likely reason is due to an effect on the BRB, because this would involve a change in the morphology of the tight junctions and in recent years these have been found to be very flexible. Shen and colleagues[14], working with membranes in the kidney, identified two types of protein, one fairly immobile, the other dynamic. One immobile type, claudin-1, remained stably localized in the tight junction. Another type, occludin, diffused rapidly within the tight junction. A third type, zonula occludens-1, also highly dynamic, moved between the membrane and the cytoplasm. These results show that the tight junction has a flexible morphology and this probably means that the membrane in which it lies has a variable permeability. It must be supposed that the agents affecting the BRB interact in some way with some of these proteins. There are estimated to be 30 proteins attached to tight junctions, so the possibilities are very large. It would certainly improve the treatment of macular edema if more was learned about the molecular biology of the BRB.

Recently, the drawback due to the loss of the vitreous has been overcome by using an implant consisting of the drug embedded in a biodegradable polymer base, injected into the posterior segment via a 22-gauge needle[15-19] As far as I know the only drug used in these implants has been dexamethasone (Ozurdex: Allergan Pharmaceuticals) and some good results have been obtained, achieving peak concentrations of dexamethasone at 2 months and continued release up to 6 months[15]. However, in one report in which the dexamethasone implant was used to treat central retinal vein occlusion (CRVO), neovascular glaucoma (NVG) developed within six months[20]. It was uncertain to what extent the NVG was due to the CRVO or to the implant. Nevertheless, there does not seem to be any reason why other drugs should not be incorporated into a similar implant.

The vitreous is an interesting material. The cells in the ciliary body that make it in the embryo degenerate after birth, so when the vitreous is removed it is not restored.

However, using stem cells it might be possible to recreate the vitreous either in vitro or in vivo and this might provide a better environment for the implant. Alternatively, it should not be difficult to make an artificial vitreous and place it in the posterior segment.

## CONCLUSION

Macular edema can be created by several ocular diseases and disorders and attempts to correct it have also made use of several methods, often unsuccessfully. Two such methods are described here: hyperbaric oxygen and estrogen. These two methods are effective while being applied but the effect is lost when the treatment is discontinued. Although in the short term the edema may be caused by a vascular disorder, the more serious and lasting edema is probably due to a breakdown in the blood-retina barrier (BRB) and this is more difficult to cure. Research into the mechanism of the tight junctions in the BRB may lead to a solution to this problem.

## ACKNOWLEDGMENTS

I thank my ophthalmologist, Assoc Prof. Alex P Hunyor, for his kind attention over many years, for performing the operation to remedy the macular hole in my left eye. I thank the staff at the Retina Associates, Chatswood, NSW, Australia, for their efficient treatment of my visual problems. I am very grateful to Dr Michael Bennett and the staff at the Department of Diving and Hyperbaric Medicine, Prince of Wakes Hospital, Sydney, NSW, Australia for arranging and conducting me through the HBO sessions in the hyperbaric chamber.

I thank Clive Jeffrey and John Dodson for excellent technical assistance with the illustrations.

## REFERENCES


[1] Campbell AJ and Hill L. Concerning the amount of nitrogen gas in the tissues and its removal by breathing almost pure oxygen. *J. Physiol.*, 1931; 71: 309-322.

[2] Chen J and Smith LEH. Retinopathy of prematurity. *Angiogenesis,* 2007; 10: 133-140.

[3] Oguz H. and Sobaci G. The use of hyperbaric oxygen therapy in ophthalmology. *Surv. Ophthalmol.,* 2008; 53: 112-120.

[4] Noell WK. Visual cell effects of high oxygen pressures. *Fed. Proc.,* 1955; 14: 107-108.

[5] Chang Y-H, Chen P-L, Tai M-C et al. Hyperbaric oxygen therapy ameliorates the blood-retinal barrier breakdown in diabetic retinopathy. *Clin. Exp. Ophthalmol.,* 2006; 34: 584-589.

[6] Carlisle R, Janphier EH and Rahn H Hyperbaric oxygen and persistence of vision in retinal ischemia. *J. Appl. Physiol.,* 1964; 19: 914-918.

[7] Anderson B Jr, Saltzman HA and Heyman A. The effects of hyperbaric oxygenation on retinal arterial occlusion, *Arch. Ophth.,* 1965; 73: 315-319.

[8] Haddad HM and Leopold IH. Effect of hyperbaric oxygenation on microcirculation: use in the therapy of retinal vascular disorders. *Invest. Ophthalmol.,* 1965; 4: 1141-1149.

[9] Krott R, Heller R, Aisenbrey S and Bartz-Schmidt K-U. Adjunctive hyperbaric oxygenation in macular edema of vascular origin. Undersea Hyperbar M . 2000; 27: 195-204.

[10] Jansen EC and, Nielsen NV. Promising visual improvement of cystoid macular oedema by hyperbaric oxygen therapy. *Acta Ophthalmol. Scand.,* 2004; 82: 485-486.

[11] Davey DF, Ng P and Burke W. A novel method for determining regional visual acuity in man and its application to a case of macular hole. *J. Neurosci. Methods,* 2004 138: 113-122.
[12] O'Donnell ME, Lam TI, Tran LQ, et al. Estradiol reduces activity of the blood-brain barrier Na-K-Cl cotransporter and decreases edema formation in permanent middle cerebral artery occlusion. *J. Cereb. Blood Flow Metab.,* 2006; 26:1234-1249.
[13] Pfaffenrath V. Efficacy and safety of percutaneous estradiol vs placebo in menstrual migraine. *Cephalalgia,* 1993; 13: 244.
[14] Shen L, Weber CR and Turner JR . The tight junction complex undergoes rapid and continuous molecular remodeling at steady state. *J. Cell Biol.,* 2008; 181:683-695.
[15] Chang-Lin J-E, Attar M, Acheampong AA, et al. Pharmacokinetics and pharmacodynamics of a sustained release dexamethasone intravitreal implant. *Invest. Ophthalmol. Vis Sci.,* 2011; 52: 80-86.
[16] Chang-Lin J-E, Burke JA, Peng Q, et al. Pharmacokinetics of a sustained–release dexamethasone intravitreal implant in vtrectomized and nonvitrectomized eyes. *Invest. Ophthalmol. Vis Sci.,* 2011; 52: 4605-4609.
[17] Boyer DS, Faber D, Gupta S, et al. Dexamethasone intravitreal implant for treatment of diabetic macular edema in vitrectomized patients. *Retina,* 2011; 31:915-923.
[18] Reibaldi M, Russo A, Zagari M, et al. Resolution of persistent cystoid macular edema due to central retinal vein occlusion in a vitrectomized eyefollowing intravitreal implant of dexamethasone 0.7 mg. *Case. Rep. Ophthalmol.,* 2012; 3:30-34.
[19] Merkoudis N, Granstam E. Treatment of postoperative cystoid macular oedema with dexamethasone intravitreal implant in a vitrectomized eye – a case report. *Acta Ophthalmol.,* 2013; 91: e238-e239.
[20] Joshi L, Tomkins-Netzer O, Menezo V, et al. Dexamethasone implants and neovascular glaucoma in central retinal vein occlusion. *Acta Ophthalmol.,* 2013; 91: e239-e240.

# INDEX

## A



## B

## E



## F



## G

## K



## L



## M



## N

## O



## P



## Q



## R

## U



## V